Understanding
SPORTS
MASSAGE

Patricia J. Benjamin, PhD
Chicago School of Massage Therapy

Scott P. Lamp
Southeastern Sports Massage

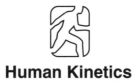

Human Kinetics

Library of Congress Cataloging-in-Publication Data

Benjamin, Patricia J., 1947-
    Understanding sports massage / Patricia J. Benjamin, Scott P.
Lamp.
        p.   cm
    Includes bibliographical references and index.
    ISBN 0-87322-976-2
    1. Massage therapy.   2. Sports physical therapy. I. Lamp, Scott
P., 1956- . II. Title.
    RM721.B476   1996
    615.8'22'088796--dc20   95-49158
                                        CIP

ISBN: 0-87322-976-2

Acquisitions Editor: Richard A. Washburn, PhD
Developmental Editor: Larret Galasyn-Wright
Managing Editor: Julie Marx Ohnemus
Editorial Assistants: Karen Grieves and Coree Schutter
Copyeditor: June Waldman
Proofreader: Julia Anderson
Indexer: Theresa Schaefer
Typesetter and Layout Artist: Francine Hamerski
Text Designer: Stuart Cartwright
Cover Designer: Keith Blomberg
Cover Photographer: Wilmer Zehr
Illustrator: Viki Marugg
Printer: Versa Press

Printed in the United States of America   10 9 8

Human Kinetics
Web site: www.humankinetics.com

United States: Human Kinetics, P.O. Box 5076, Champaign, IL 61825-5076
800-747-4457
e-mail: humank@hkusa.com

Canada: Human Kinetics, 475 Devonshire Road, Unit 100, Windsor, ON N8Y 2L5
800-465-7301 (in Canada only)
e-mail: hkcan@mnsi.net

Europe: Human Kinetics, P.O. Box IW14, Leeds LS16 6TR, United Kingdom
+44 (0) 113 278 1708
e-mail: humank@hkeurope.com

Australia: Human Kinetics, 57A Price Avenue, Lower Mitcham, South Australia 5062
08 8277 1555
e-mail: liahka@senet.com.au

New Zealand: Human Kinetics, P.O. Box 105-231, Auckland Central
09-523-3462
e-mail: hkp@ihug.co.nz

This book is dedicated to my teachers at Mother McAuley Liberal Arts High School, who taught me about academic excellence and the joy of sports, and to Helen M. Heitmann, who has been an inspiration to me throughout my professional career.

PJB

This book is dedicated to Benny Vaughn, ATC, and Sue Lewis, PT, who contributed greatly to my understanding of health care.

SPL

CONTENTS

PREFACE

Sports massage is becoming a familiar component in the training routines of Olympic and professional athletes, as well as in school and university sports programs, at health clubs, and on the sidelines of various competitive events. It enriches conditioning programs, helps athletes prepare for and recover from competition, reduces the potential for injuries, and aids in injury rehabilitation. Ultimately, sports massage enhances performance.

Although massage was commonly used by trainers and athletes in the first half of the 20th century, it had virtually disappeared from the sports scene in the United States between 1950 and 1980. Except for sports massage specialists, those who have hands-on involvement with today's athletes tend to have little knowledge or skill in this time-honored practice.

Athletic trainers and sport physical therapists, who share in the history of sports massage, have found their niche in the prevention, treatment, and rehabilitation of injuries. They may use massage in a limited way as one of many rehabilitation modalities. Sports massage specialists, on the other hand, use their highly developed manual skills to apply massage in the context of the whole athlete for general health maintenance and performance enhancement.

Because sports massage includes nonmedical applications, coaches and athletes themselves can use simple techniques. Self-massage and giving massage to another athlete are easy to learn.

The purpose of this book is to show sport professionals how to incorporate sports massage into their athletes' training and health care programs. This book is written for coaches, athletic trainers, sport physical therapists, and sport physicians and chiropractors interested in learning more about sports massage and how it benefits athletes. It will also interest massage practitioners who specialize in sports massage.

This text discusses the nature of sports massage, its theoretical and scientific underpinnings, and its varied applications. Scientific and experiential evidence is presented in the context of the whole athlete to help explain the positive physiological and psychological effects of massage. Historical vignettes reveal a rich tradition of massage for athletes.

On the practical side, individual sports massage techniques are described in detail along with the use and intended effects of each. We include many suggestions and ideas on ways that coaches and athletes can use massage.

We also explain the finer points of planning and giving a massage and discuss body mechanics, palpation, technique selection, movement qualities such as rhythm and pacing, monitoring pain, and the massage routine.

A special feature of the book is a chapter on how to implement a sports massage program in various settings and how the sports massage specialist can cooperate with other sport and health professionals to provide the best possible care for athletes.

This book is written primarily for sport professionals and, therefore, assumes an existing knowledge base in basic sport science. We hope you find it useful for understanding how sports massage can enhance your athletic program.

ACKNOWLEDGMENTS

The authors would like to thank all those who gave their encouragement and support to this project. Special thanks go to sports massage therapists Patricia Archer, Jill Bielawski, Robert King, Marge MacLeod, Nikki Nicodemus, and Benny Vaughn for sharing their expertise and suggestions for the book; to Richard van Why for unearthing valuable historical information; to Victoria Carmona for thoughtful critiques, encouragement, and photography; to Alicia Davis, Deb Doricchi, Martha Griffin, Rick Haesche, and Susan Taff from the Connecticut Center for Massage Therapy for their help in preparing illustrations; and to the countless athletes and sports massage specialists who have kept the tradition of sports massage alive and added to its body of knowledge over the years.

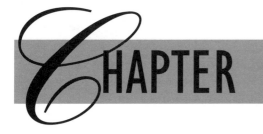

CHAPTER 1

INTRODUCTION TO SPORTS MASSAGE

A coach kneading an athlete's shoulders before an event, a trainer frictioning a player's calves during a time-out, a sport physical therapist using deep-transverse friction for rehabilitation, and a massage therapist stroking and kneading tired legs at a marathon finish line—these are all examples of the use of massage to improve athletic performance. Similar scenes have occurred in sports arenas since ancient times and attest to the enduring value of massage for athletes in a variety of situations.

In this book we will explore the many applications of massage in various sports settings, describe commonly used techniques, and discuss the theory behind the practice. We will present simple massage techniques and applications that coaches and athletes can use every day. Athletic trainers and sport physical therapists will learn ways to use massage not only to treat injuries but also to enhance performance. Massage therapists will find a comprehensive survey of the current theory, techniques, and applications of sports massage.

The term *massage* means to manipulate the soft tissues of the body. *Sports massage* is a more specific term to describe the science and art of applying massage and related techniques to ensure the health and well-being of the athlete and to enhance athletic performance.

THE MANY USES OF MASSAGE IN SPORTS

A coach may knead an athlete's shoulders prior to competition for any one of several reasons. The coach may be attempting to relieve muscular tension caused by physical conditions (e.g., splinting due to soreness) or by anxiety. She or he may also be reassuring the athlete by using touch, thereby relieving anxiety and facilitating greater focus. A coach may use massage as one of many methods to bring out the athlete's best performance.

Athletic trainers and sport physical therapists typically use massage for rehabilitation in the tradition of physiotherapy. In this context, massage is only one of many modalities for treating injuries. Massage is often an effective treatment for conditions such as tendinitis, strains, sprains, and adhesions.

The athlete may use self-massage for general conditioning, to loosen a tight muscle, to facilitate stretching, or to prepare emotionally for an event. Athletes can learn to use simple massage techniques on each other.

The five major applications of massage in sports are listed below. The first three applications are restorative (i.e., their goal is to return the athlete to optimal condition), and the last two are related to the athlete's training and competition schedule.

- Recovery—To enhance the athlete's physical and mental recovery from strenuous sports activity

- Remedial—To improve a debilitating condition

- Rehabilitation—To facilitate healing after a disabling injury

- Maintenance—To enhance recovery from strenuous exertion, to treat debilitating conditions, and to help the athlete maintain optimal health

- Event—To help the athlete prepare for and recover from a specific competitive event. Event massage is divided into three subapplications.

  1. Pre-event—To help prepare the athlete mentally and physically for a specific event

  2. Interevent—To help the athlete recover from a specific event while preparing for an upcoming one

  3. Postevent—To help the athlete recover from an event and either administer first aid or refer problem conditions to another health professional

Resurgence of Sports Massage in the 1970s to 1990s

Interest in the use of massage for training athletes was rekindled in the United States in the 1970s after a 20-year hiatus. Its comeback resulted from several factors.

Sports massage regained credibility among runners when Lasse Viren, the "Flying Finn," set a world record time in the 10K and an Olympic record in the 5K at the 1972 Summer Olympics in Munich. Runners learned that Viren received deep massage daily—a discovery that sparked interest in sports massage in the United States. Its use by other high-profile individuals also called attention to the value of massage for serious athletes.

Sports massage has been highly visible at international events. Professional massage therapists have organized and staffed services at many recent Olympic Games, including the 1984 Summer Olympics in Los Angeles, California, and the 1988 Winter Olympics in Calgary, Canada. At the 1988 Summer Olympics in Seoul, Korea, the U.S. Track and Field Team traveled with their own sports massage specialists.

Since its first appearance at the Boston Marathon in 1985, the National Sports Massage Team (NSMT) of the American Massage Therapy Association (AMTA) has provided pre-event and postevent massage at many national and international games, including the 1987 Pan-American Games in Indianapolis, Indiana, and the 1990 Goodwill Games in Seattle, Washington. The NSMT will provide sports massage at the 1996 Summer Olympics in Atlanta, Georgia.

In addition, local AMTA sports massage teams work at local and regional events, such as community fun runs. The AMTA Connecticut Chapter offered sports massage at the Special Olympics World Games in Connecticut in 1995.

Athletes at all levels are discovering the benefits of massage, with interest growing among professional athletes and sports teams. Several teams employ a traveling sports massage specialist, and many individual professional athletes have their own massage therapists.

Amateur athletes, weekend warriors, and fitness participants see massage as an aid to their training programs, helping them to continue their workouts with less stiffness and soreness. Participants now recognize the relaxation and stress reduction that massage brings, this service being an important adjunct to fitness programs.

The resurgent interest in sports massage has been fueled by the re-emergence of therapeutic massage as a profession, which has spurred a growing number of trained massage practitioners. Sports massage has become a popular specialty among massage therapists. It is available today to athletes of all skill levels, in private offices, in training rooms, at finish lines, and at most modern health clubs.

THE SPORTS MASSAGE SPECIALIST

Massage is the primary focus of one type of sport professional, the sports massage specialist. Because massage is useful for many general and specific purposes, experts in massage are valuable members of the athlete's support team. Their specific role is to apply massage and related techniques in order to ensure the health and safety of athletes and to enhance their performance.

How do sports massage specialists function in the sport setting? Their role can be best understood using the coaching model. Coaches interact with their athletes on a regular basis; they set practice and training routines, teach and fine-tune technique, give encouragement, and guide athletes through competitions. Coaches work with the unique talents and physical abilities of each athlete to elicit the best possible performance.

H. Joseph Fay and the International Sports Scene in 1916

H. Joseph Fay, an Australian authority on massage for athletes, described the use of massage in international sports in 1916. In his book, *Scientific Massage for Athletes*, Fay notes how popular massage was among winning athletes from the United States, and he rejects the recurring argument that the benefits of massage for athletes may be overestimated.

On arrival in this country [England] I was surprised to hear that massage, or rubbing as it is wrongly called, was not considered to be beneficial to the athlete, and that work on the ordinary exercise lines was quite sufficient to get a man in any branch of athletics.

This statement in the face of the continued American successes in the big international meetings of the amateur world seemed to lack weight, for it was generally known that the American athlete was decidedly keen on having his rub after exercises—in fact that it formed quite as important a part of his training as his work on the track.

Again, it was no news that the Swedes had adopted American methods of training which included massage, their coach having got his experience of athletics in the United States. Even the success of the Swedes at the last Olympiad did not convince the English athletic world. (p. 15)

Fay attributes the English attitude that massage for athletes was a waste of time by explaining that the English version of rubbing was too light—a "tickling"—and that it lacked system. He says, "When I saw the attempt I understood the expressions of the great English multitude who objected to it" (p. 16). Fay further defines scientific massage for athletes:

What is massage as those countries know it who have been successful in international contests?

It is the systematic treatment of muscle not lightly but vigorously to bring about definite results. These are: 1. To rid the muscle of waste or poisonous substances which are collected in its depths, and which bring about fatigue and stiffness. 2. To produce additional growth of bone and muscle. . . . (pp. 17-18)

The difference between an average trainer and a practical one is that the former merely pats or plays with the hide, while the latter works the meat, or muscle, between the hide and the bone so that it is in its highest state for exercise. (p. 20)

Fay's book contains some interesting information about the techniques and scope of sports massage in the early 20th century. He described massage techniques in three main groups: friction, kneading, and vibration. Fay refers to the "electric effect of the masseur," electricity being transferred from the trainer to the athlete. Although he considered the case for electricity "largely overdone," his account reveals that some early 20th-century trainers believed in what now is called *energy* work (p. 26).

Moreover, Fay's section on treating sprains with massage and applications of cold shows that the scope of sports massage extended to some rehabilitation (pp. 61-68).

Although coaches cannot guarantee a winning performance, the appropriate use of time-tested coaching methods can increase the athlete's performance potential. The actual performance is a complex phenomenon—not easy to explain—but clearly influenced by the coach.

Sports massage specialists share the coaches' goal: to increase performance potential. They use massage in various situations to support the health and well-being of the whole athlete and ultimately to enhance performance. Sports massage specialists are most effective when they build strong bonds with an athlete and become part of the athlete's support team.

The value of sports massage has traditionally been defined in broad terms that include psychological as well as physiological factors. Sports massage is concerned with the whole athlete.

THE WHOLE-ATHLETE MODEL

The *whole-athlete model* acknowledges that athletes bring the totality of their lives to their sports participation. The old metaphor of the athlete as a machine (i.e., the mechanist model) must yield to the more organic view of the whole athlete in order to clarify the role of massage in enhancing sport performance.

In the whole-athlete model, the sports participant is seen as an organic system, a complex of physical, emotional, mental, and social factors that interact with an external environment (see Figure 1.1). The quality of an athletic performance is the result of the synergistic interaction of the parts of the whole system.

Central to the whole-athlete concept is the idea that a change in any one part of the system affects the organism as a whole. For example, on the purely physical level, all tissue and systems are intimately connected and, therefore, affected by the health and activity of all other tissues and systems. This is especially true for systems that pervade the body, such as the integumentary, nervous, circulatory, lymphatic, and musculoskeletal systems, and the connective tissue that binds them all.

In addition, changes in physical condition affect the mental and emotional state, and vice versa. An increasing amount of medical research has clearly established this connection (Workshop on Alternative Medicine, 1994). In sports, for example, muscular aches and pains may disturb an athlete's mental focus, and anxiety may cause muscle tension that interferes with fluid movement.

The athlete's relationships with other athletes, coaches, team physicians, athletic trainers, sports massage therapists, and other sport and health care professionals are also important components of the system. These relationships can have a profound effect on the mental, emotional, and physical state of the athlete, on the group dynamics of the sport setting, and, therefore, ultimately on sport performance.

External factors in the sport environment such as training and competition schedules, traveling, facilities, and equipment are also important to consider. To complete the picture, we must add family and friends, school and work, and even community, national, and global situations to our systems concept of the whole athlete.

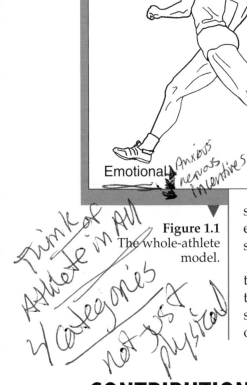

Figure 1.1 The whole-athlete model.

CONTRIBUTIONS OF SPORTS MASSAGE

Massage has been used for various purposes by different sport professionals, and it is perhaps because massage works on so many levels (i.e., physical, mental, emotional, and social) that it has been found to be a useful tool in addressing the whole athlete.

Exactly how does sports massage enhance athletic performance? Sports massage, applied skillfully, increases performance potential in three major ways. Sports massage

- optimizes positive-performance factors while minimizing negative ones,

- decreases injury potential, and

- supports soft tissue healing.

Sports massage helps to optimize positive-performance factors such as healthy muscle and connective tissues; normal range of motion; high energy; fluid and pain-free movement; and mental calm, alertness, and concentration. It can help minimize negative-performance factors such as dysfunctional muscle and connective tissue, restricted range of motion, low energy, staleness, pain, and high anxiety.

Positive-performance factors are enhanced over a period of time with regular maintenance massage. Pre-event and interevent massage provide a last minute tune-up just before performance.

Sports massage also decreases injury-potential factors. It is most effective in helping to prevent acute injuries resulting from abnormal tissue conditions (e.g., muscle tears in tight muscles) and chronic injuries caused by wear and tear (e.g., tendinitis).

One of the most basic benefits of regular sports massage comes from the routine and direct palpation of soft tissues. The massage giver can monitor subtle changes in the condition of tissues and locate potential trouble spots during massage before the athlete becomes consciously aware of them.

Especially in the case of chronic injury, an athlete will feel pain with the pressure applied during massage before the injury is far enough along to elicit pain in the absence of pressure. Thus massage can uncover injuries at the subclinical level that can be dealt with before they get to the clinical stage.

When an injury does occur, the sports massage specialist joins the entire health care team in helping the athlete recover. The goal is to help the injury heal as quickly and effectively as possible and to minimize side effects and the possibility of reinjury.

Massage can facilitate soft tissue healing in a number of ways. It helps reduce both primary edema and the possibility of secondary injury caused by the pressure of increased fluid in the area of trauma. Increased circulation resulting from massage can move healing nutrients to the injury site. Massage can also promote the creation of strong and mobile scar tissue and prevent and break adhesions in the injured area and surrounding tissue.

Sports massage enhances athletic performance through the effects of specific massage techniques performed alone and in combination, both at the time of application and accumulated over a period of time. In addition, the interaction of the therapist and the athlete can have important effects. Understanding just how sports massage works is the subject of the remainder of this chapter.

SCIENTIFIC RESEARCH

There are abundant testimonials about the benefits of sports massage from enthusiastic athletes and plenty of anecdotal evidence to support its use for training and competition. But explaining *why* massage seems to enhance athletic performance is a challenge. Although the question seems simple, the answer is as complex as the athletes who engage in sports.

What does research tell us about sports massage? There is a limited amount of research dealing directly with sports massage; however, many studies have been done on the effects of massage in general. These studies taken together, and in the context of the whole athlete, offer some understanding of how sports massage enhances athletic performance.

Unfortunately, much of the recent research on sports massage has been based primarily on the mechanistic model with a focus on pre-event applications. Although this approach has brought some understanding of sports massage, it is narrow in scope and limited in its ability to explain the more complex phenomenon of the whole athlete. For example, some skeptics have based their doubts about the benefit of sports massage as a whole on narrow experimental studies of pre-event or warm-up massage (Boone, Cooper, & Thompson, 1991; Harmer, 1991). These studies tested the effects of pre-event massage as if it were a "pill," which administered once would magically improve performance. Not surprisingly, the researchers found little effect.

In addition, sports massage research has done little to acknowledge the mind–body connection. In fact, athletes have been cautioned that "the recuperative benefits [of sports massage] may be more psychological than physiological" (Boone, Cooper, & Thompson, 1991, p. 51). In the whole-athlete perspective, the interplay of the mind and body cannot be ignored without severely limiting our understanding of human performance. The psychological effects of massage, the subtle effects of touch itself, and the relationship between the person performing the massage and the athlete have also been ignored or discounted.

Kresge (1983) offers further explanation of the limitations of experimental research to account for the effectiveness of sports massage.

It has been frequently noted that clinical results of massage are often more dramatic than experiments with massage would indicate. Massage, however, tends to have a cumulative effect that is not shown in short-term experiments. It is a science and art combining a variety of strokes in infinite ways to best suit individual situations, while scientific experiments must employ standardized, repeatable procedures. (p. 370)

Cumulative effects over time, the uniqueness of each application of sports massage to a specific athlete, and the characteristic synergy of sport performance make it difficult to design and carry out valid experimental research showing a simple cause-and-effect relationship of massage to sport performance.

Contrary to the teachings of the mechanistic model, massage specialists are admonished to

resist the tendency to focus our attention upon localized and objectively predictable *effects*, and must always strive to include ever broadening and more complexly interrelated *processes* in our ways of thinking and working. . . . Whatever we do with our hands must be done with the knowledge clearly in mind that all of the physical and mental elements within the human being are inextricably related. (Juhan, 1987, p. 90)

With the whole athlete in mind, we will proceed to look at research that studies the various physiological and psychological effects of massage and propose a theory of how they combine to enhance athletic performance. Beyond its simple predictable effects, the ultimate and most powerful influence of massage on actual athletic performance depends on how it is applied and integrated into the total athletic experience.

CONSTELLATION OF EFFECTS

Sports massage techniques produce a constellation of primary ondary effects that may have either an immediate influence oɪ. ρeгtor- mance or accumulate over time. These effects cannot be explained in a neat, concise, linear fashion, but are best viewed as complex interrelated phenomena. However, to begin to understand what is happening, we will use the metaphor of a chain reaction.

In this chain reaction, sports massage techniques induce primary ef- fects (e.g., improved blood circulation) that bring about secondary effects (e.g., better cell nutrition, faster recovery) that optimize positive- performance factors (e.g., by allowing for longer and more intense prac- tice) and, thereby, ultimately increase performance potential. For example, greater elasticity of connective tissue may lead to greater range of mo- tion and greater power, thereby enhancing performance; or the relax- ation response may reduce precompetition anxiety and lead to better concentration and better performance.

These simplified examples show the progression of effects. Several sec- ondary effects may result from one primary effect of massage. For ex- ample, increase in blood circulation (primary effect) can also increase removal of retained metabolites, decrease edema, and hasten repair of microtraumas (secondary effects). Table 1.1 shows examples of impor- tant primary and secondary effects of sports massage.

These primary and secondary effects interact in complex ways. The constellation of effects occurs in the context of the whole athlete and therefore interacts with other factors such as coaching, training, and the competition schedule. In order to apply sports massage for the best re- sults, practitioners must understand as much as possible about each primary and secondary effect, their relationships to each other, and their influence on the athlete's health, well-being, and performance.

Table 1.1 | **Important Primary and Secondary Effects of Sports Massage**

Primary effects refer to the physiological and psychological condition of the athlete and include

- improved fluid circulation,
- muscular relaxation,
- general relaxation,
- functional separation of muscle and connective tissue,
- formation of strong mobile scar tissue,
- connective tissue normalization,
- increased mental alertness and clarity, and
- deactivation of trigger points.

Secondary effects refer to performance-related outcomes and include

- greater energy,
- greater flexibility and range of motion,
- fluid movement,
- faster recovery,
- pain reduction, and
- appropriate level of emotional stimulation.

Practitioners must also be skilled in choosing and performing the techniques that will bring about the desired effects based on the needs of each athlete.

Primary Effects

The primary effects of massage include its influence on various physiological and psychological functions of the body and mind and on the condition of specific tissues. Some of the primary effects of particular interest in sports massage include improved blood and lymph circulation, muscular and general relaxation, functional separation of muscle and connective tissue, formation of strong mobile scar tissue, connective tissue normalization, increased mental alertness and clarity, and deactivation of trigger points. These effects are called *primary* because they effect the physiological and psychological condition of the athlete.

It is important to remember that the general term *massage* refers to a variety of techniques that differ widely in their application and effects. A specific massage technique or combination and sequence of techniques might have one effect, but a different technique, combination, or sequence might produce a totally different effect. The specific effects of each massage technique are described in greater detail throughout the book.

Improved Fluid Circulation

Improved blood and lymph circulation are perhaps the most recognized primary effects of classic Western massage. Research has consistently demonstrated the increase in lymph flow in normal tissues during massage (Yates, 1990).

Similarly, increase in blood circulation is a well-accepted result of massage. However, there are different theories about the mechanism involved. Increased circulation may result from the direct physical and mechanical effects on the vessels, circulatory changes resulting from the release of vasodilators, or changes elicited by reflex responses of the autonomic nervous system stemming from tissue stimulation (Yates, 1990). We suspect that variations of massage techniques (e.g., light or deep gliding strokes, compression, or percussion) work through different mechanisms to produce the same result, that is, increased circulation.

Muscular Relaxation

That massage induces muscular relaxation is a well-accepted premise. It occurs when a hypertonic muscle returns to normal muscle tone or even to a temporarily flaccid state.

Muscle relaxation may also be the result of several different mechanisms and is often a neuromuscular phenomenon directly related to the athlete's psycho-emotional state. Muscular relaxation may be the result of changes in the autonomic nervous system as part of a general relaxation response that will be discussed in the next section. It may also result from a conscious letting-go of muscle tension by higher brain centers, which occurs when an athlete assumes a passive role in letting the

practitioner freely move soft tissue and joints. In this cas€
cilitates a response similar to the relaxation techniques of au
ing and progressive relaxation.

Yates (1990) postulates that muscle relaxation may also be
to the increased sensory stimulation that accompanies mass͏

> Whenever a change occurs in a sensory input to a spinal cord seg-
> ment, an increase or decrease in motor activity within that segment
> will follow unless rapid compensatory adjustments are made. Mas-
> sage causes a massive increase in sensory input to the spinal cord,
> so widespread readjustments in these integrated reflex pathways
> can be expected. It seems reasonable that such a perturbation would
> spontaneously result in renormalization of imbalances of tonic ac-
> tivity between individual muscles and muscle groups. Thus, where
> hypertonicity has developed in a specific muscle, relative to other
> muscles, in response to a sustained posture or an emotional state
> but persists beyond its original cause, the effectiveness of massage
> may be due in part to increased sensory stimulation. (pp. 11-12)

The concept of *functional unity* of the musculature as explained by Juhan
(1987) is also important. Muscles are commonly described as separate
anatomical units, but their functioning is best understood as an intricate
interplay of muscular tension and release, with synergistic and antagonistic
relationships among muscle compartments throughout the entire body.

> That is to say that if I pull on any part of a woven fabric, I create a
> pull over the entire warp and woof. . . . We almost never find a
> single discreet muscle that is tense. Rather, we will find areas of
> tension, or body-wide patterns of tension, whose boundaries do
> not necessarily follow the anatomical divisions of muscle compart-
> ments. And we will never release [relax] a single muscle, but rather
> we will increase a *range of motion* that involves several, or many,
> separate compartments. (Juhan, 1987, p. 113)

General Relaxation

Although general relaxation is listed here as a primary effect, it is actually a complex phenomenon encompassing many different aspects. The
concept of body–mind interaction is essential to understanding this response. The well-known relaxation response may be induced either by
calming the mind first, followed by physiological changes (psychoso-
matic), or by relaxing the body first, followed by psychological changes
(somatopsychic). Decreased tone of the sympathetic nervous system and
increased tone of the parasympathetic nervous system trigger the physiological responses. The relaxation response includes a decrease in oxygen
consumption, heart rate, respiration, and skeletal muscle activity and an
increase in skin resistance and alpha brain waves (Curtis, Detert, Schindler,
& Zirkel, 1985).

An interesting aspect of the relaxation response, like the stress response,
is that the characteristics are so interrelated that inducing one will tend
to reflexively kick off the others. For example, slow, deep breathing is
commonly used to induce the relaxation response. Muscle relaxation can

[handwritten margin note: one thing affects the other... think]

have the same effect and is doubly effective when supplemented by diaphragmatic breathing.

It is the slow, smooth, gliding movements of massage that trigger the relaxation response. It should come as no surprise that massage is particularly effective on the back (Field et al., 1992; Yates, 1990).

Functional Separation of Muscle and Connective Tissue

The separation of muscle and connective tissue is achieved through the simple mechanical action of lifting and broadening, as well as by applying a more focused shearing force across the parallel organization of muscle fibers. This action breaks connections or adhesions made between muscle, connective (fascia, tendon, ligament) tissues, and other tissues, "unsticking" any gluing that would inhibit fluid movement. Kneading, deep-transverse friction, and broadening techniques are most effective for muscle fiber and connective tissue separation.

Formation of Strong Mobile Scar Tissue

During the remodeling, or scar-maturation, phase of soft tissue healing, massage can provide the mobilization needed to create a strong yet supple scar. During scar formation, collagen fibers are first arranged randomly to form a weave or patch to repair tissue damage. At a later stage, the scar begins to rearrange itself along the direction of stress or line of pull of the muscle.

The mechanical action of deep-transverse friction helps produce a scar with more parallel fiber arrangement and fewer transverse connections that limit movement. James Cyriax, a well-known champion of deep friction, reasons that the best way to break interfibrillary adhesions is by forcibly broadening the tissues, which is best accomplished through deep-transverse friction. This application is effective for all connective tissue, including muscles, tendons, and ligaments (Cyriax & Cyriax, 1993).

Connective Tissue Normalization

As the most pervasive tissue in the body, connective tissue can have a profound effect on the ability of the body to move. It is found most prominently in ligaments and tendons and also in fascia around and within the musculature. It possesses a property called *thixotrophy* by which it can become "more fluid when it is stirred up, and more solid when it sits without being disturbed" (Juhan, 1987, p. 68).

Under chronic stress or chronic immobility, connective tissue tends to thicken and become rigid, lose its range of movement, and through its interconnectedness with surrounding and even remote tissues inhibit movement overall. The chronic stress of intense training can have this effect. Massage is ideal to remedy this situation.

> By means of pressure and stretching, and the friction they generate, the temperature and therefore the energy level of the tissue has merely been raised slightly. This added energy in turn promotes a more fluid ground substance which is more sol and ductile, and in which nutrients and cellular wastes can conduct their exchanges

more efficiently. . . . Skillful manipulation simply raises energy levels and creates a greater degree of sol (fluidity) in organic systems that are already there but are behaving sluggishly. (Juhan, 1987, pp. 69-70)

The formation of abnormal collagenous connective tissue, called *fibrosis*, is curtailed with massage techniques of kneading, deep friction, and other passive movements (Yates, 1990). This is most likely the result of maintenance of a more fluid ground substance combined with the prevention and breaking of adhesions.

Increased Mental Alertness and Clarity

Certain massage techniques, particularly fast-surface (skin) friction, kneading, and percussion, stimulate the organism and elicit the alertness necessary for competition (Birukov & Peisahov, 1979). That they are most effective when performed with speed and lightness attests to the response as coming from stimulation of the tactile nerve endings in the skin. This bombardment of sensory data is a "wake-up call" to the brain.

A job stress study conducted by the Touch Research Institute at the University of Miami in Florida confirms the value of massage for increasing mental alertness. Subjects receiving a 20-minute massage in a chair twice weekly for a month reported less fatigue and demonstrated greater clarity of thought, improved cognitive skills, and lower anxiety levels. EEG, alpha, beta, and theta waves were also altered in ways consistent with enhanced alertness (Field, Fox, Pickens, Ironsong, & Scafidi, 1993).

Deactivation of Trigger Points

Travell and Simons (1983) define trigger points as

a focus of hyperirritability in a tissue that, when compressed, is locally tender and, if sufficiently hypersensitive, gives rise to referred pain and tenderness, and sometimes to referred autonomic phenomena and distortion of proprioception. Types include myofascial, cutaneous, fascial, ligamentous and periosteal trigger points. (p. 4)

In addition to pain, trigger points may be accompanied by restricted range of motion, weakening of the maximum contractile force of an affected muscle, and tension of muscle in the immediate vicinity. Firm digital pressure is recommended to deactivate trigger points (Travell & Simons, 1983). This could take the form of deep-stroking massage, kneading, or simple, direct thumb pressure (see "Trigger Points" on page 52).

Secondary Effects

The secondary effects of sports massage are performance-related outcomes of the primary effects. For example, the prevention and breaking up of adhesions (primary) leads to more pain-free and fluid muscle movements (secondary). Improved blood circulation (primary) promotes faster recovery from heavy workouts (secondary), which permits more frequent and concentrated practice sessions.

The division between primary and secondary effects is not always sharp, but the concept is useful for describing the chain reaction that eventually leads to increased performance potential. Some of the main secondary effects of sports massage are greater energy availability, normal range of motion, more fluid movement, faster recovery, and reduced pain and anxiety.

Greater Energy

Energy is depleted and muscle fatigue sets in when the body cannot keep up with supplying nutrients and carrying away waste products from muscles in continuous contraction. Muscular contractions may occur from conscious movement on the part of the athlete and also from unconscious contractions, such as with chronically hypertonic or spasming muscles. The latter may be either the result of inadequate recovery or a sustained stress response.

Massage helps in an active way by improving circulation, which hastens the removal of metabolites and makes needed nutrients more available. Massage also helps conserve energy and prevent energy depletion through muscular and general relaxation. Thus, more energy is available to the athlete for training and competition.

Normal Range of Motion and Fluid Movement

Any number of factors may restrict movement at a joint. The factors include hypertonicity, scarring in muscle and connective tissue, adhesions, trigger points, and connective tissue thickening and rigidity. Application of appropriate massage techniques alleviates these conditions and allows a normal range of motion. The same factors that inhibit normal range of motion also affect the ability of the body to move smoothly.

A cooperative study by sport physical therapists and a massage therapist (Crosman, Chateauvert, & Weisburg, 1985) found that massage can significantly increase range of motion in the hamstrings. Increased flexibility was immediately evident and lasted for at least 7 days postmassage. The massage techniques used were effleurage (sliding strokes), deep effleurage, stretching effleurage, petrissage (kneading), and friction (deep-circular and deep-transverse).

Faster Recovery

Athletes require adequate time to recover from intense training and competition. Accumulated negative effects result in the overtraining syndrome characterized by increased frequency of injury, irritability, increased resting heart rate, altered appetite, apathy, and decreased performance (Anshel, 1991).

Sports massage addresses many aspects of recovery, including reduction of muscle soreness and stiffness caused by accumulation of metabolites, acceleration of healing of damaged tissues, relaxation and lengthening of tight muscles, and general relaxation to restore physical and emotional balance. Zalessky (1979) summarizes the restorative effects of massage in his article "Coaching, Medico-Biological and Psychological Means of Restoration."

> Under the influence of massage, blood circulation is improved; removal of wastes and toxic substances from tissues is accelerated; metabolic and oxidative processes are activated; central and peripheral nervous system activity is normalized. Massage accelerates resorption of infiltrates in muscles, ligaments and tendons; decreases muscle tension after work; increases functional neuromuscular activity.

An often quoted research study on recovery massage done at the turn of the century by Mosso and Maggiora focused on restoring work capacity in muscles. R. Tait McKenzie reported in 1915 that "there was a greater increase of working capacity after the use of petrissage than from either of the other movements [friction and percussion], but the results were obtained by using in turn all three" (pp. 338-339).

This early research on the positive effects of massage on work capacity was substantiated by a 1990 study by Jordan and Jessup at the University of North Carolina at Chapel Hill in which subjects performed a series of leg extensions on a Universal leg machine at 80% maximum until they could not continue (i.e., to extreme fatigue). The control group experienced passive rest after the leg extensions; the experimental group received a 10-minute massage.

The study compared pretest and posttest torque readings of right-quadriceps strength as measured by an isokinetic dynamometer. In the control group, strength decreased significantly, and in the experimental group strength actually increased somewhat. The recovery massage given consisted of effleurage (sliding strokes), deep effleurage, petrissage (kneading), and compression broadening (Jordan & Jessup, 1990).

The early Mosso and Maggiora research also traced the source of recovery effects of massage to improved circulation in the fatigued muscle (McKenzie, 1915). These early findings are substantiated in a more recent study of Russian athletes (Dubrovsky, 1982).

Research by McSwain (1990) compared the effects of massage, exercise, and rest on recovery after strenuous exercise by measuring the clearance rate of blood lactate. After a bout of strenuous exercise and a 5-minute interval, subjects were given either a 25-minute recovery massage (mainly sliding strokes and kneading), a 25-minute recovery exercise routine, or simply a rest period. Blood lactate levels (BLA) were measured at 5, 15, 30, and 50 minutes after the strenuous exercise.

As expected, both exercise and massage were more effective than rest for recovery. Massage and exercise were found to be equally effective for recovery (no statistically significant difference) during the period they were administered. However, the effects of massage were found to continue at a greater rate than the effects of exercise after treatment, and the massage group had the greatest percent decrease in BLA at the end of the 50-minute recovery period. Unfortunately, measurements were not taken after 50 minutes. It would have been interesting to see how long the effects of massage in decreasing BLA levels would have continued.

Based on her findings and a recommendation by Bell (1964), McSwain (1990) suggests that "a combination of exercise recovery (early in recovery), followed by massage (later during recovery) might be more effective in lowering BLA concentrations than either method of recovery alone" (p. 53). An alternative interpretation from McSwain's recovery-period chart might be that if an athlete has at least 50 minutes between events a 25-minute massage is more effective than exercise for recovery.

A number of Russian studies support the use of a combination of methods for recovery, given the time and resources. The Russians use a greater variety of recovery methods that, in addition to exercise and massage, include hydrotherapy (e.g., baths, sauna, steam room) and some physiotherapy methods (e.g., ultraviolet light, ultrasound, and electrotherapeutic procedures). All of these methods promote increased circulation and muscular and general relaxation (Birukov & Pogosyan, 1983; Matveeva & Tsirgiladze, 1985; Sinyakov & Belov, 1982; Zalessky, 1979).

Russian literature also discusses the athlete's need to return to a normal psychological and emotional state following the stress of strenuous training and competition. What they call the "psychological means" of restoration includes some familiar stress reduction and relaxation techniques termed *psycho-regulatory training* (PRT), for example, biofeedback and autogenic relaxation techniques. One article also mentions such things as lifestyle and leisure time, a friendly team atmosphere, and even selecting music and color to help achieve psychological recovery (Zalessky, 1979, 1980).

It is interesting that the Russian literature does not mention massage as a means to relaxation and stress reduction, possibly due to their emphasis on the medical or strictly physiological applications of massage. However, there is ample research to support the use of massage for such psychological recovery (see "General Relaxation" on page 11).

Pain Reduction

The pain-reduction (analgesic) effect of massage is well documented (Kresge, 1983; Yates, 1990). Simple muscle relaxation and improved circulation help relieve the pain associated with hypertonicity and the accompanying ischemia. A pain-contraction cycle induced by muscular tension may then be interrupted, thus removing the source of pain (Kresge, 1983; Yates, 1990). Massage and stretching may also relieve pain associated with myofascial trigger points. This includes pain at the site of the trigger point, satellite trigger points, and muscles that lie within the pain reference zone of a trigger point (Travell & Simons, 1983, 1992).

There has been some evidence that massage induces the release of central nervous system endorphins that modulate pain-impulse transmission. This may be the result of physical or psychological reactions to massage; however, more research is needed in this area (Yates, 1990).

It has also been proposed that massage may activate the neural-gating mechanism in the spinal cord through stimulation of large-fiber proprioceptors and cutaneous mechanoreceptors. This has been suggested as an explanation for the temporary analgesia associated with deep-friction massage in the treatment of tendinous and ligamentous injuries (Yates, 1990).

Appropriate Level of Emotional Stimulation

An appropriate level of emotional stimulation is necessary for peak performance. Low levels of emotional stimulation, as evidenced by feelings of heaviness, sluggishness, or sleepiness, impede performance as do high levels, such as that caused by competition anxiety.

Different massage techniques can help athletes achieve their optimal level of stimulation. Slow, smooth, sliding strokes have a sedative effect, and rigorous kneading, squeezing, and percussion have an energizing and vitalizing effect (Birukov & Peisahov, 1979).

CONTRAINDICATIONS AND CAUTIONS

Sports massage should be avoided in all cases where its application will worsen a problem condition. However, the concept of contraindication is not a black-and-white issue. Most problem conditions are not absolute contraindications for massage, but certain cautions may be in order.

As a general rule, massage is contraindicated and should *not* be applied in the following situations:

- Around an infection
- Near suspected fractures
- Directly over open wounds or burns
- Near undiagnosed tumors
- Over varicose veins (avoid deep pressure and movement away from the heart)
- Where blood clots or phlebitis are present or suspected
- Over a skin rash
- When contagious disease may be transmitted to the massage therapist or to the athlete

Cautions should be taken with athletes with diabetes, kidney disease, cancer, and certain cardiac conditions, such as recent heart attack and excessively high blood pressure. In these cases the athlete's health care provider should be contacted for any specific directions.

Caution is also in order for persons with cold and flu symptoms, as well as any others reporting "not feeling well." Massage may worsen such conditions and cause nausea. During postevent sessions, watch for signs of dehydration and hyperthermia or hypothermia. Do not attempt sports massage until these conditions have subsided.

Extreme caution should be taken during remedial applications of sports massage (e.g., with edema, strains, sprains, and tendinitis). The massage therapist should not hesitate to refer the athlete for medical assessment when there is any doubt as to the severity of the condition.

Massage has been used effectively as part of the treatment for inflamed tissues and joints. However, great care must be taken, and massage should be accompanied by inflammation-reducing modalities.

Care should always be taken to choose appropriate techniques and apply them correctly for the situation at hand. Certain conditions may be worsened by one massage technique but respond very well to another. In order to apply massage safely and effectively, the practitioner should know the effects of each technique and its correct application.

Chapter 2 describes in detail the basic techniques used in sports massage, identifies the effects of each technique, and makes suggestions for their use with athletes.

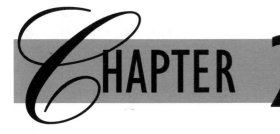

CHAPTER 2

TECHNIQUES AND BASIC SKILLS

Individual massage techniques form the building blocks of a sports massage session. The skilled practitioner must blend these techniques together into a smooth, flowing sequence and perform them with a certain rhythm, pace, and pressure to produce the specific physiological and psychological effects of sports massage.

The techniques presented here are manual, that is, they are performed by hand. The human hand can be a very precise instrument. It is capable of sensing myriad bits of information about the condition of the tissues it is touching and of performing techniques with both gross and finely coordinated movements.

To achieve the desired results, the massage giver must understand the physiological and psychological effects of each technique and its variations. One of the more subtle aspects of massage is that varying the rhythm, pacing, and pressure of a technique will produce different effects.

The techniques described in this chapter are largely derived from classic Western massage (e.g., Swedish and Russian massage) that is the basis for most sports massage used in the West today. We also mention some techniques from other forms of massage therapy, for example, acupressure and trigger point work.

In the following sections, we give detailed descriptions of the basic techniques of sports massage. As in all manual arts, each practitioner will modify, and apply in a slightly different way, the techniques presented here as his or her own unique style evolves with practice and experience.

HAND AND FINGER PLACEMENT

For a clear understanding of how to apply the techniques of massage, it is essential to consider the various positions of hand and finger placement. We will identify and describe the most commonly used hand and finger placements in the following section.

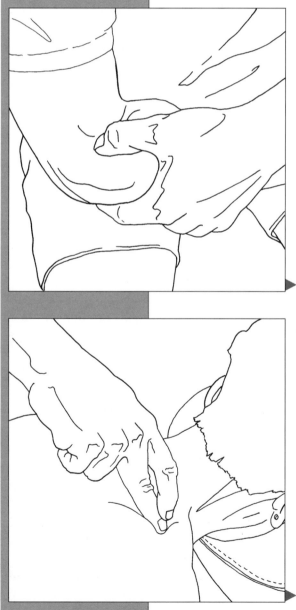

Single-Digit Placement

In single-digit placement, the tip or the pad of a single finger or the thumb applies the massage technique. The rest of the hand may touch the athlete, but the massage movement comes from a single digit. Figure 2.1 shows that single-digit placement is very effective for reaching the tendinous attachments associated with tennis elbow, especially in self-massage.

▶ **Figure 2.1**   Single-digit placement.

Single-Digit Overlay

Single-digit overlay is the single-digit placement supported by the use of another digit of the same or other hand. One finger applies the massage while another is placed on top of the first to assist with strength and coordination of the massage movement (see Figure 2.2).

▶ **Figure 2.2**   Single-digit overlay.

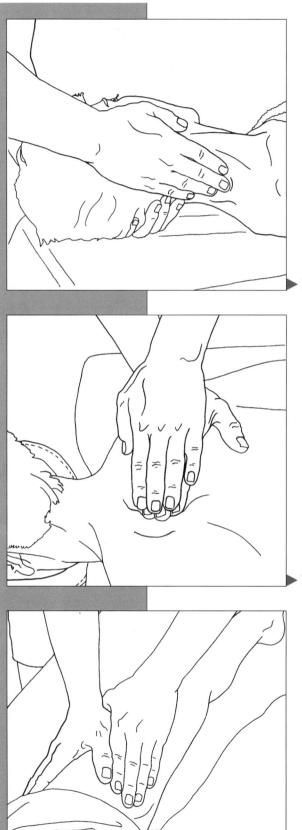

▶ **Figure 2.3** Multiple-digit placement.

Multiple-Digit Placement

In multiple-digit placement the tips or the pads of several fingers or both thumbs apply the massage. Figure 2.3 demonstrates that multiple-digit placement is effective for massaging a longer portion of muscle in a single sweep, especially in hard to reach areas like the back of the neck.

(CASTANETS)

Multiple-Digit Overlay

In multiple-digit overlay, shown in Figure 2.4, the fingers of one hand apply the massage while the fingers of the other hand are placed on top of the first to assist with strength and coordination of the massage movement.

Shoulder circles

▶ **Figure 2.4** Multiple-digit overlay.

Full-Palmar Placement

For full-palmar placement, the entire palmar surface of one or both hands, including the digits, is in contact with the body part to be massaged. This broad contact surface is appropriate for techniques that move bodily fluids and is illustrated in Figure 2.5.

BASIC - 1-2 LOW BACK

▶ **Figure 2.5** Full-palmar placement.

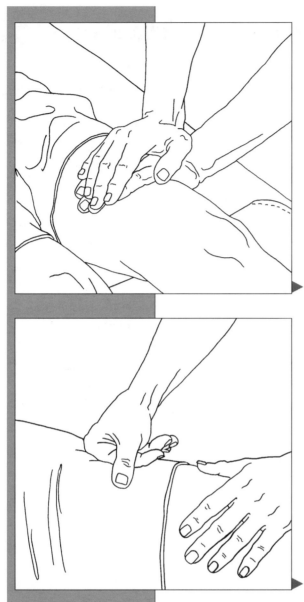

Full-Palmar Overlay

The entire palmar surface of one hand applies the massage while the palm of the other hand is placed on top of the first to assist with strength and coordination of the massage movement. This placement is especially useful for working on large, well-muscled areas and facilitates the pressure needed to be effective in such areas. Figure 2.6 shows this placement at work on the muscles of the thigh.

▶ **Figure 2.6** Full-palmar overlay.

Knuckle Placement

The dorsal surface of the proximal phalanx bones performs the massage when the hands are in the knuckle placement. The entire length of the bone makes contact, not just the knobby joints. This placement is not with a tight fist, which is rigid and unyielding, but is performed with a loose fist, which allows for some resilience upon the application of pressure. Figure 2.7 shows the contact surface in proper knuckle placement.

▶ **Figure 2.7** Knuckle placement.

MASSAGE TECHNIQUES

Sports massage techniques are based on classic Western massage, which historically includes the five technique categories of effleurage, petrissage, tapotement, friction, and vibration. The approximate English equivalents to the French terminology used in sports massage today are, respectively, sliding movements, kneading, percussion, friction, and vibration.

Each of these five categories includes many technique variations. Some of these variations are applied for specific effects and are important enough in sports massage to warrant their own names; for example, sliding movements such as thumb slides and broadening and compression. Some newer techniques such as positional release have also been incorporated into sports massage. Adjunct techniques used in sports massage include joint range of motion, joint mobilizations, and stretching.

Palpation skills, while not techniques as such, are important in the application of massage. It is through palpation skills that the giver of massage assesses the condition of the tissues, an assessment that helps in choosing which techniques to use.

The remainder of this chapter describes in more detail the most common techniques used in sports massage and explains their general applications.

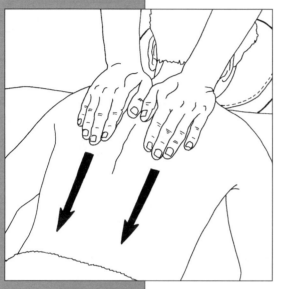

Figure 2.8
Sliding movement on the back using full-palmar placement.

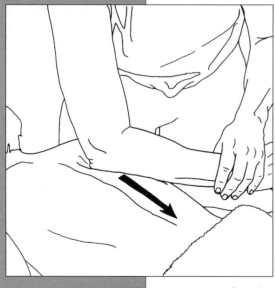

Figure 2.9
Sliding movement on the back using the elbow.

Sliding *FUll BACK - HEART*

Sliding movements are very effective, easy to learn, and have numerous variations and uses. They are the most frequently used massage movements. They involve sliding across the skin with steady pressure and are best applied with some form of oil or cream lubricant to reduce friction. However, oil may not be needed if the technique is performed lightly, with little pressure.

Figure 2.8 depicts the most common sliding-movement technique where the hands conform to the body part using the full-palmar position and the entire palmar surface is in contact with that part. Hands remain somewhat relaxed in order to maintain conformity throughout the movement. Apply a long sliding motion along the length of the part with steady pressure throughout. If the part includes a bony prominence, such as the patella, the pressure may be released during that portion of the movement. After the sliding motion covers the length of the body part, move your hands back to the starting point by sliding superficially over the surface of the skin.

Variations of the basic sliding movement are achieved by simply changing the hand placement to any of those described earlier in this chapter, the direction of the movement, the amount of pressure, or by using another body part such as the elbow or the forearm (see Figure 2.9). With experience you can create many variations of this movement.

Faltering effleurage, a sliding movement found in Russian-style massage, actually has a stimulating effect, in addition to warming the tissues. This technique as taught by Zhenya Wine of the Kurashova Institute is performed by alternating hands in swift, short, brushing slides over the skin (see Figure 2.10). The hands are held stiffly, and the rhythm is uneven (i.e., stroke, stroke, pause). This change in the length and rhythm of the movement changes its effect on the nervous system.

Sliding movements can be performed with a broad contact surface (see Figure 2.8) using considerable pressure, and they are very effective at moving bodily fluids. Thus they may be used to enhance circulation to areas where injury or immobilization may restrict blood flow. After intense physical activity, or after a period of immobilization,

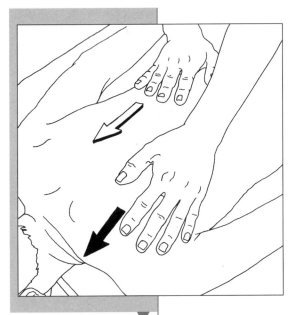

Figure 2.10
Faltering effleurage—a
brisk sliding movement
alternating hands for a
stimulating effect.

1-2 moves

body tissues often retain metabolites. Sliding movements can reduce the metabolites by flushing out tissues through increased circulation.

In fact, sliding movements may benefit the healthy circulatory system by enhancing normal venous return. Massaging toward the heart, or in the direction of venous return, logically will assist in the movement of stale, low-oxygen blood out of an area and the subsequent replacement of oxygen-rich blood into the area.

It is important to note that when sliding movements are applied to the extremities using heavy pressure, the motion must be distal to proximal in order to avoid possible venous damage. Athletes with a history of phlebitis or blood clots should not have their extremities massaged with heavy pressure, as the pressure could mechanically dislodge a clot. Also, any type of inflammation or edema caused by infection is a contraindication for massage. In fact, massage may help spread the infection mechanically.

Techniques that use sliding movements may reduce edema (an abnormal accumulation of fluid within tissue) not associated with infection or acute inflammation. When there is swelling of the distal extremities, such as with a sprained ankle, sliding movements applied to the extremity can aid in the movement of the edemic fluids away from the ankle and encourage healing, oxygen-rich blood into the area. When edema is present, it is very important to perform sliding movements with great care; incorrect application increases the risk of further injury.

Sliding movements may also facilitate the movement of lymphatic fluid toward the lymph nodes where foreign substances are filtered out. It is important to note, however, that some types of cancer are spread via the lymphatic system. There is some concern that the effect of massage on the lymphatic system may contribute to the spread of such cancers; therefore it is important to consult the attending physician before beginning any massage program on an athlete with cancer.

In addition to their mechanical effects on body fluids, sliding movements can also have a soothing effect on the nervous system. This effect is produced when sliding movements are performed in long, slow applications and repeated at a steady rhythmical pace. Performed in this fashion and with extremely light pressure, this technique will reduce neurosensitivity in situations of acute pain. For example, the athlete with a minor cervical injury often exhibits a great deal of associated muscle spasm, voluntary and involuntary splinting, and apprehension toward treatment. Sliding movements applied with little pressure, in a steady rhythm, will not only reduce the neurosensitivity in the area, but will also produce relaxation in underlying muscle tissue. In addition, the soothing effect of the technique will reduce psychological apprehension. By reducing apprehension and relaxing the underlying muscles, these techniques may prepare the athlete for other forms of therapy.

While performing techniques with sliding movements, the fingers search for differences in tissue consistency, pliability, and response to pressure. In this way, sliding movements are a useful evaluation tool and provide more comfort to the patient than the standard palpation exam.

In the context of a massage session, sliding movements also work as a transition from one massage technique to another or as a soothing movement after a less comfortable technique has been applied.

Sliding is a multipurpose and variable massage movement that primarily affects the blood and lymph circulation, nerves, muscles, and emotional well-being and comfort of the athlete.

Thumb Slide   *Bridge*

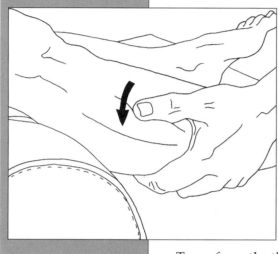

Figure 2.11
Thumb slide on the tibialis anterior using single-digit placement.

Sliding the thumb along a specific muscle while applying heavy pressure is called a *thumb slide*. This technique differs from general sliding movements in that its effect is very specific, it has little effect on general circulation, and is not used to reduce hypersensitive nervous tissue. The purposes of the thumb slide are to reduce muscle hypertonicity, increase muscle elasticity, and improve muscle elongation potential. Thumb slides also provide slight spot-specific passive muscle stretching, which make them very valuable on areas that are difficult to stretch effectively like the tibialis anterior on the front of the shin. Thumb slides across the tissues of the tibialis anterior are shown in Figure 2.11.

To perform the thumb slide place your thumbs in the single-digit, overlay, or multiple-digit position. Apply a sliding motion with even pressure along the length or across the width of the part being massaged. This technique is typically performed with very deep pressure and has a strong mechanical effect on muscle and fascial tissues. Use the distal segment of the thumb for best pressure and repeat the action several times in a single direction.

Broadening   — *Low Back stretches — cross fibers*

The sliding-movement technique referred to as *broadening* has its primary effect on broadening the muscle belly, but may also be applied to tendons and fascial tissues. Broadening refers to any sliding technique that involves a compression of muscle and fascial tissues followed by a sliding motion in a direction that broadens the tissue.

For large muscles or groups of muscles, place your hands on the body part in full-palmar position, with the heels of the hands meeting in the center of the muscle being massaged (see Figure 2.12). Apply sufficient pressure to compress the tissues, while moving the palms out and away from one another in a direction transverse to the length of the muscle fibers. The focus of the pressure is to the heel of the hands. Repeat the process along the body part until the entire part has been massaged. For smaller muscles the thumbs move in a similar fashion (see Figure 2.13).

The application of broadening techniques enhances the ability of the muscle to broaden, which may enhance the contractibility of that muscle and perhaps even enhance muscle strength. A muscle's strength lies in

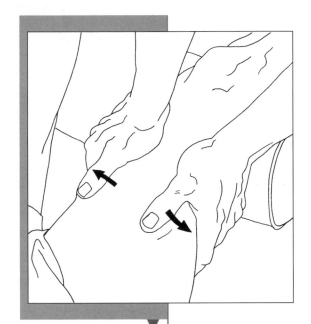

Figure 2.12
Broadening technique
on the quadriceps
using full-palmar
placement.

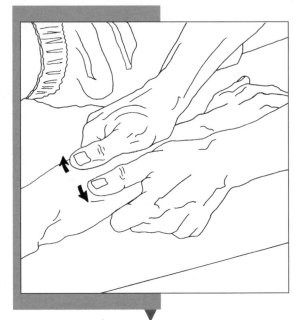

Figure 2.13
Broadening technique
on the forearm using
the thumbs.

its ability to contract. When a muscle contracts, it shortens and becomes broader. If a muscle becomes hard from fascial build-up, its ability to broaden during contraction may be compromised. Hypertonic muscles, especially those from chronic conditions, feel hard and ropelike. Tissue in this condition may not perform optimally and is more likely to suffer injury. A muscle in good condition should feel firm yet elastic, not hard, and flat or broad rather than round and ropelike. The technique of broadening can assist in restoring the muscle to its natural broadening potential.

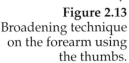

Kneading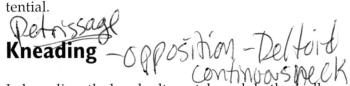

In kneading, the hands alternately and rhythmically squeeze, lift, and release the muscle. Kneading is typically performed on groups of muscles rather than on an individual muscle and is applied to the belly rather than the tendons of those muscles. Basic kneading begins with the hands in full-palmar position.

When massaging larger muscle groups such as the quadriceps, use two-handed kneading. First squeeze and lift with one hand and then with the other in a rhythmical and alternating fashion as shown in Figure 2.14. Repeat the movement in different places along the muscle belly with a moderate tempo. Take care not to pinch the skin or adipose tissue while performing this technique.

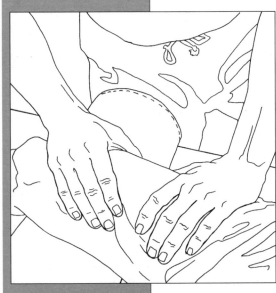

Figure 2.14
Kneading using two
hands.

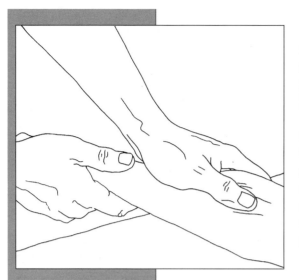

Figure 2.15
Kneading using one hand with other hand supporting.

Use one-handed kneading to massage a smaller muscle group such as the wrist extensors. Figure 2.15 shows how to use one hand to support the body part to be massaged and the other hand to squeeze and lift the muscle belly.

As the technique progresses, note the warming of the tissue and increasing muscle elasticity. Kneading produces passive muscle movement and a slight muscle stretching and results in increased local circulation and reduced muscle hypertonicity. As an evaluative technique, kneading can help you determine the general elasticity of any given muscle group.

Percussion

Tapotement — wrists, loose as possibile

Percussion is the general term for a variety of techniques that apply rapid, rhythmic, percussive movements to the body with the hands or fingertips. Figure 2.16 shows the rapid movement of percussion.

Six percussion techniques are in common use, and each has its own descriptive name:

- Beating — *fists*
- Hacking
- Slapping — *finger tips*
- Cupping —
- Pincement —
- Tapping — *finger tips*

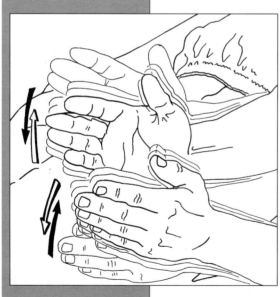

Figure 2.16
Rapid movement of percussion.

All variations are performed in a similar fashion, but each technique uses a different striking surface. The athlete perceives a slightly different sensation from each technique, but the end result is the same: physiological and psychological stimulation.

Each technique of percussion creates a unique sound, depending on the way the hand strikes the body. These sounds contribute to the psychologically stimulating effect of the technique and to the enjoyment of receiving percussion.

Percussion can enhance an athlete's sense of "readiness" for practice or competition. The use of several different varieties one after another and intermixed is most pleasant and beneficial.

To apply percussion techniques successfully, it is essential to perform the movements with relaxed hands and fingers and to begin the movements at the elbows. While the left hand strikes the body part, the right hand is in the air. The right hand then comes down to strike while the left hand lifts off the body part. Repeat this action in rapid and rhythmical succession.

Percussion may be performed over any muscled part of the body, but is not typically performed over bony prominences or in any area where soft tissue may be harmed, such as over the kidneys or the abdominal cavity.

In spite of the aggressive, unskilled, and often painful depiction of percussion in cinema and television productions, properly performed percussion is actually quite delightful and invigorating to receive. These rapid and rhythmical techniques require significant practice to be applied with skill. Some people simply lack the rhythm needed and, unfortunately, never become proficient at performing percussion. Figures 2.17 through 2.22 show the six common percussion techniques.

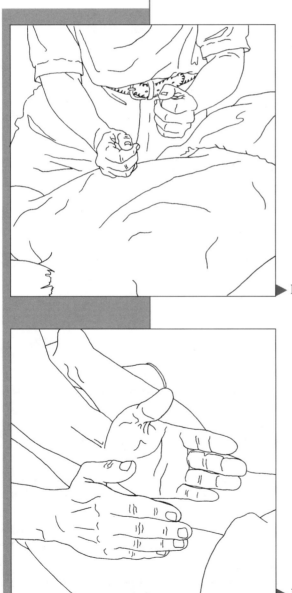

Beating

The hands are in a lightly closed fist using the hypothenar eminence and the small finger as the striking surface. The wrist is loose, rather than rigid, during the movement so that the effect is not jarring to the recipient.

▶ **Figure 2.17**   Beating.

Hacking

The hands are held with the palms facing one another and the fingers relaxed in slight flexion. The fifth digit (small finger) is more flexed than the fourth; the fourth more flexed than the third, and so on. The small finger and the tips of the third and fourth fingers act as the striking surface. The wrist and fingers remain loose during the movement.

▶ **Figure 2.18**   Hacking.

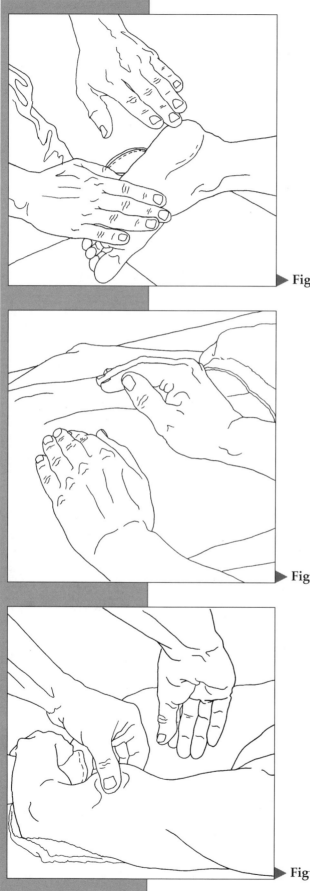

Slapping

The hands are held with the palms toward the part to be massaged. Use either the entire palmar surface or just the pads of the fingers to lightly slap the area.

Figure 2.19   Slapping.

Cupping

The hands are held so that the thumb and fingers are pressed together and slightly flexed with the palmar surface becoming concave and forming a cup. The striking surface is the outer rim of the "cup," consisting of the small finger, thumb, fingertips, and the heel of the hand. The center of the palm does not make contact.

Figure 2.20   Cupping.

Pincement

The hands are held with palms toward the part to be massaged. The thumb and fingers are used to lightly pick up the tissue. Perform this motion rapidly but not aggressively.

Figure 2.21   Pincement.

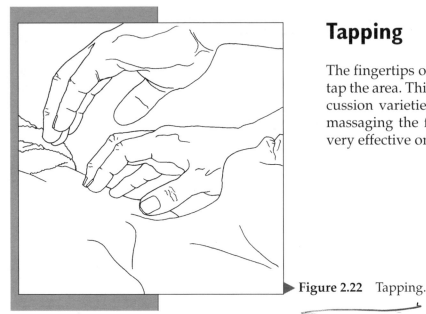

Tapping

The fingertips or the pads of the fingers lightly tap the area. This is the most delicate of the percussion varieties and is typically reserved for massaging the face and head. Tapping is also very effective on the chest.

Figure 2.22 Tapping.

Friction

Friction is one of the oldest known massage techniques, and it has been mentioned in medical and health texts since ancient times. One trainer in the early 20th century remarked, "When in training after running and perspiring freely one should subject the skin to harsh friction from course towels" (Pollard, 1902). Friction is often used to increase blood flow to the skin, causing a warming effect; it is quite natural to rub yourself briskly when you feel cold.

The Rubdown

Athletes at the turn of the century were quite familiar with the *rub-down*. A rubdown consisted mainly of superficial skin friction with the hand or with various objects, such as a brush, horsehair glove, or coarse towel. In 1902 Pollard reported the thoughts of different trainers about a rubdown's benefits:

> Oxford athletes are never allowed to do cross country running without first rubbing their legs with horsehair gloves or with hands. . . . After sweating, sponge with hot saltwater. Dry with a coarse towel, then use horsehair glove freely. . . . The best remedy for congestion and labored breathing is a glass of warm brandy and plenty of hard friction on the feet, legs and thighs. . . . In all cases vigorous rubbing should follow the use of water; a bath attendant who knows something about massage is invaluable, for how to rub down a man or a horse is an art. (p. 21)

Michael C. Murphy (1914), a well-known trainer and early Olympic track coach, considered the rubdown a must for athletes. He described a self-administered rubdown, which he advised doing daily after an early morning bath:

The bath should be followed by a vigorous rub-down. . . . After the body has been dried thoroughly the massage should begin with the feet, and every part of the body should be vigorously rubbed, at least five minutes being taken for the operation. The massage movement is very simple and consists merely of rubbing the hands vigorously over the skin with a circular motion. The back can be rubbed as well as the legs and arms by using a rough towel and drawing it back and forth vigorously. This sort of rub-down will be a splendid tonic for the skin, and at its conclusion the body will glow from the blood flowing to every part as nature intended it should. (pp. 6-7)

Frequently a bath attendant with little training gave the rubdown, done with variations in Turkish baths, public baths, and athletic clubs as a general health measure. Stafford complained, "Indiscriminate 'rubbing' and rough manipulation . . . forms, in too many cases, the bulk of the athletic trainer's armamentarium" (1928, p. 8). Rubdown came to mean a superficial, nonspecific, low-skill massage.

Because the rubdown took place in a bath and locker-room environment and looked like a massage to the untrained eye, it was often confused with the more specific and skillful massage done by a trained practitioner. In *Athletic Training Methods* (1925), Mat Bullock of the University of Illinois wrote, "The beneficial effects of a good massage are so important that it should not be confused with that anathema of the author—'rub down.' The conscientious trainer's language does not include the word, rub down, which is entirely too light and frivolous an expression of massage" (p. 15).

The term *rubber* is found in early writings to refer to a person who gives massage, regardless of the type, including the rubdown and more skilled forms of massage. In describing the treatment for sore shins, for example, Murphy states that "if the runner has the services of a trainer and rubber he will be properly cared for" (1914, p. 161).

Friction for the purpose of superficial warming is applied with any of the various hand placements and by moving over the surface of the skin in rapid back and forth movements creating friction between your hands and the athlete's skin as shown in Figure 2.23.

Friction applied to the deeper tissues is very specific in its application and is therefore performed with a small contact surface, using either the thumb or the fingertip(s) placed in single-digit, single-digit-overlay, multiple-digit, or multiple-digit-overlay position. The movement of deep friction consists of short, brisk strokes applied in either circular or back-and-forth motions. Apply sufficient pressure so the digit does not slide across the surface of the skin but rather the skin and the digit move together as a unit (see Figure 2.24), ensuring a frictioning effect on the tissues beneath the skin.

Deep frictioning prepares the environment for recovery by stimulating the rush of oxygen- and nutrient-rich blood into the area and has the added mechanical effect of breaking or reducing adhesions in muscle

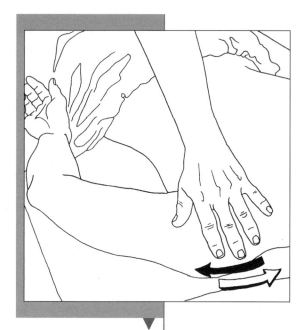

Figure 2.23
Superficial warming
friction.

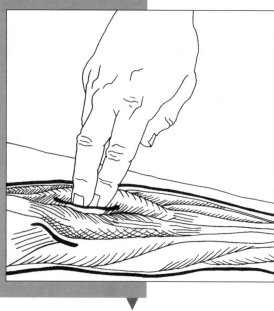

Figure 2.24
Deep friction.

and fascial tissues. These effects account for friction's particular value
when applied around articulations, tendinous attachments, or the site of
a healed injury. One of the most commonly applied techniques of deep
friction is called *circular friction*.

Circular Friction

Circular friction is applied in a circular direction covering an area typically no more than 1 square inch. It
is performed with a single digit or by using the same
digit of both hands. Continuous, rhythmical repeti-
tions give the overall impression of a single movement.

When both hands are used, the circular movements
are performed simultaneously and in opposite directions (see Figure 2.25). The left and right thumb
are placed in close proximity to each other on the
body. Simultaneously, the left thumb creates a coun-
terclockwise motion while the right thumb creates a
clockwise motion. The thumbs arrive back at the
starting places synchronically.

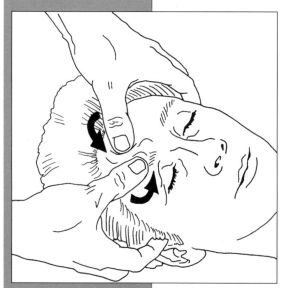

Figure 2.25
Circular friction using
the thumbs.

Deep-Transverse Friction

Deep-transverse friction is the technique most commonly applied either to reduce the amount of scar tissue or to create a more pliable
scar at an injury site. The therapist wishing to work with sport injuries will need to be well versed in this technique.

Postinjury scars form in a haphazard manner with scar fibers overlapping one another in all directions. This results in a matting effect that adheres muscle fibers to each other and to bony structures. A problem often occurs when extensive scarring limits the muscle's ability to contract and broaden. Also, a site of chronic pain or inflammation may develop in areas where normal tissue joins scar tissue that is unable to accommodate the changes in tension during muscle activity.

Deep friction breaks down the scar between neighboring fibers while it leaves intact the scarring that reconnects a damaged fiber to itself. This action promotes the formation of a pliable, small scar that does not unnecessarily adhere to other muscles or bony surfaces and allows the muscle to broaden sufficiently. These effects reduce the potential for injury at the site of the scar.

In the *Illustrated Manual of Orthopedic Medicine*, Cyriax and Cyriax (1993) present some basic principles of using deep-transverse friction to treat muscle and tendon lesions. These principles include the following:

- Friction must be given deeply with digit and skin moving together.
- Administer friction to the precise site of the lesion.
- The friction effect is paramount, not the pressure.
- Position the athlete to render the lesion accessible and to put the tissue being treated into appropriate tension.
- A total of 6 to 12 sessions of 20 minutes each on alternate days is usually required for best results.

A muscle receiving massage must be relaxed so that the massage can penetrate deeply. A tendon with no sheath may also be in relaxed position. However, in cases of tenosynovitis, the sheathed tendon must be taut to provide a surface on which the sheath may be rubbed.

Some massage professionals believe that pain is an additional essential component of the deep-transverse friction technique. We have found that this pain exists as long as unnecessary adhesions exist. The treatment becomes less painful once the adhesions begin to mobilize. Massaging with techniques that cause pain requires special skills and considerations (see "Optimal Therapy Zone" on page 97).

In addition to working on scar tissue formation and specific injuries, deep-transverse friction can also help to heal tendinitis and tenosynovitis conditions.

Vibration

Vibration techniques apply a trembling motion with the hand or fingertips. Vibration is most commonly applied with a very light touch, but considerable pressure may also be used.

A light touch affects the superficial neuroreceptors. The fingertips assume a multiple-digit position, or the hand assumes a full-palmar position, and rest lightly on the skin. Create a small tremulous vibration movement that starts at your elbow or shoulder (see Figure 2.26).

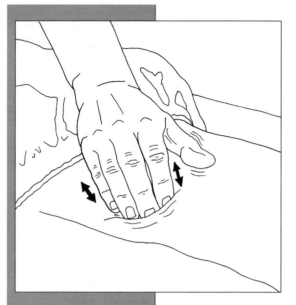

Figure 2.26
Vibration using
multiple digits.

Perform vibration with repeated applications along a body part or as one extended application while the hand slides along a body part. Apply the same technique with deeper pressure to affect the deep neuroreceptors.

Therapists use vibration to soothe nervous tissue, particularly when they treat peripheral neuritis. In cases of severe pain, light vibration may facilitate the reduction of painful impulses so that sliding or compressive massage movements may be applied.

Vibration takes much practice to master. Tappan (1988) observed that, "Vibration should not be used at all if one has not put the time and effort into learning to do it well. Done well it can be extremely soothing, but done poorly it will only cause frustration and impatience on the part of both patient and operator" (p. 91).

Vibration is one massage movement that may be performed better by machine if the vibration is to be done for a long period of time. There are many good mechanical and sound vibration devices on the market.

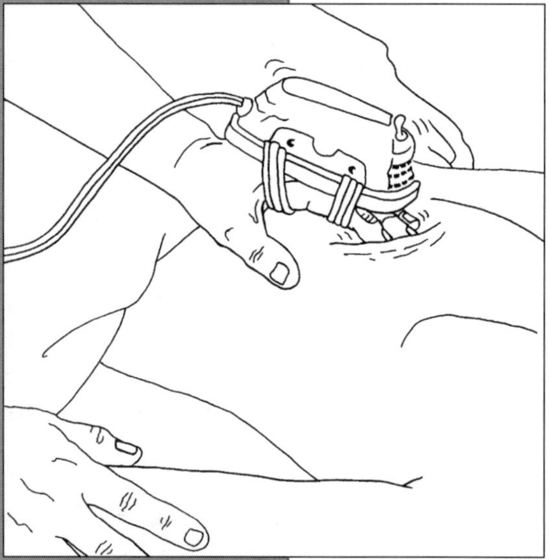

An old and effective method is to use a vibration device strapped to the back of the hand as shown in Figure 2.27. Other massage movements, such as friction, may be performed while the hand is vibrating. The soothing vibration may allow the friction to be applied more deeply.

This technique is of great value when applied to athletes suffering from hypersensitivity following an injury. It is, therefore, important for the sports massage practitioner to take time to become proficient in vibration techniques.

Manual Compression

Manual compression refers to techniques that employ a compression of tissues followed by a reduction of pressure. The most common types of compression used in sports massage are *palmar compression* and *digital compression*. Compression techniques affect local circulation, and each specific type of compression also has its own unique purpose.

Figure 2.27
Vibration using a
device strapped to the
back of the hand.

Palmar Compression

Palmar compression is applied with the hands placed on the body part in palmar-overlay position. Use your own body weight to repeatedly compress and reduce the tissue beneath the heel of the hand. The motion, as

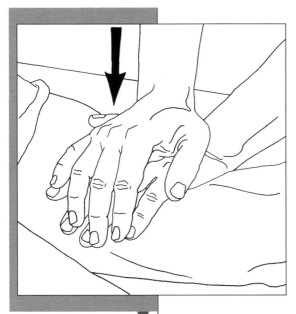

Figure 2.28
Palmar compression.

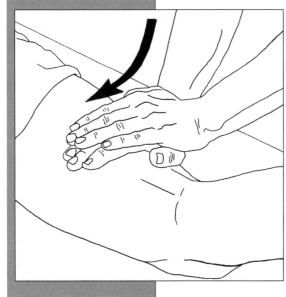

Figure 2.29
Rocking compression.

shown in Figure 2.28 is to pump straight up and down and press the muscle into the underlying bone.

Perform palmar compression slowly and with greater pressure to reduce muscle tension or spasm, to create a site-specific stretch, or to positively affect muscle elongation potential. Apply palmar compression with faster paced movement using a medium amount of pressure to warm and invigorate an athlete prior to activity.

Applying palmar compression improperly can greatly stress the wrists, causing soreness and injury. Wrists should be kept as straight as possible during the compression movement. When using palmar overlay, do not place the top hand too close to the wrist, since the pressure applied by that hand will transfer straight to the wrist and cause it to hyperextend. Pointing the fingers in the same direction will also help decrease hyperextension of the wrist (see Figure 2.28).

Vary palmar compression by changing the straight up-and-down movement to one in which the tissues are pushed slightly away from the therapist as the tissues are compressed (see Figure 2.29). This variation is called *rocking compression* because it is performed with a rhythmical motion that gently rocks the body part during the application of the compression.

Digital Compression

Digital compression is a simple technique performed with the thumb, fingertips, or elbow with sufficient pressure to compress the tissues underneath. It may be applied repeatedly along a body part or as one prolonged application to a specific site.

The point-specific pressure probably overstimulates the nerve receptors at that location, thereby temporarily "turning them off" and producing a relaxation response in the muscle tissue. Digital compression is used to deactivate trigger points, hold tender points in strain–counterstrain, stimulate acupressure and shiatsu points, and relieve stress 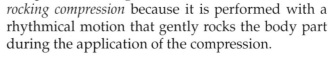 points; it is also used in other forms of "point" work (Meagher, 1990; Nickel, 1984; Travell & Simons, 1983, 1992).

It should be noted that acupressure and shiatsu are often performed in sports massage without therapists having a full knowledge of Chinese medicine; they are applied more on a basis of "for this effect, press here" (Namikoshi, 1985; Nickel, 1984). Acupressure and shiatsu are considered energy approaches in terms of theory, but they are applied using variations of basic massage techniques, particularly digital compression.

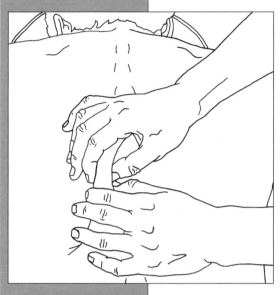

Figure 2.30
Skin rolling.

Skin Rolling

Skin rolling increases skin pliability and improves circulation to the skin and its underlying superficial tissues. It is very effective in enhancing circulation to generally tight areas such as the back.

Simply pick up the skin and gently pull it up and away from muscle tissue. There are several ways to move from one spot to another along the skin. You may use two hands moving sequentially from one spot to another, or you may alternate hands moving along an area of skin. If the skin is fairly loose, you may stay in contact and roll the skin along using the thumbs to push the skin up against the fingers as shown in Figure 2.30.

The whole area being worked should be warmed properly before performing skin rolling, and the movement should be performed slowly at first. Skin rolling may be painful if superficial circulation is poor and the tissues are adhering to each other.

APPLICATION OF TECHNIQUES WITH ACTIVE MOVEMENT

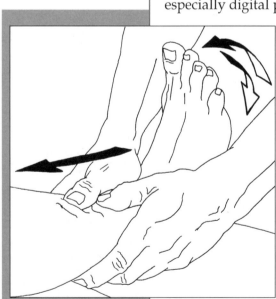

Figure 2.31
Thumb slide during active movement.

Active movement by the athlete may enhance some massage techniques, especially digital pressure, thumb slides, and broadening.

Instruct the athlete how much and how fast to contract the muscle or move the part to be massaged. (This may be best communicated by demonstration or by moving the part for the athlete.) The athlete moves as instructed while you apply the technique. Coordinate your hand movements with the movement of the athlete in order to apply the technique during the contraction.

Active movement enhances the effects of the massage technique. For example, the muscle broadens when it is contracted, and broadening the tissue during muscle contraction enhances the application of a broadening technique.

Similarly, the effects of a thumb slide may be enhanced when applied during active movement. Figure 2.31 demonstrates the application of thumb slides to the tibialis anterior tendon and the inferior extensor retinaculum combined with active movement of the ankle. This technique will not only assist in the reduction of hypertonic muscle tissue but will also assist in the proper movement of the tendons through the retinaculum. This technique is particularly appreciated by gymnasts and other athletes whose ankles repeatedly endure sudden compressive force.

ADJUNCT TECHNIQUES

In addition to the manual massage techniques, adjunct therapies may facilitate the desired response. Adjunct therapies include ice and heat therapy, hydrotherapy, or other methods that do not involve the actual manual manipulation of tissues.

Joint Range of Motion and Mobilization

Joint range of motion (ROM) refers to the active or passive movement of a joint for evaluative purposes versus joint mobilization that is done by the therapist for therapeutic benefit.

ROM is performed by actively or passively moving an articulation through its complete movement pattern. Active range of motion refers to movement that athletes perform solely by using their own muscle power; passive movement is movement that the therapist performs as the athlete relaxes.

ROM serves as an evaluative tool to determine if an injury is structural (involving the joint itself) or functional (involving the muscles responsible for the movement of that joint). It is important for the sports massage therapist, or anyone else who works with minor muscular complaints, to know how to use ROM as an evaluation tool. Athletes often misinterpret the extent of an injury: What may present as a "muscle pull" may actually involve the joint itself. If there is any indication of structural problems, immediate referral to an orthopedist for complete diagnosis is essential. If the condition presents as a muscle–tendon problem, ROM movements will provide information regarding the flexibility of that muscle.

After treatment for muscle spasm or hypertonicity, we can once again perform ROM to judge the progress. Demonstrated results help establish a positive healing mindset.

The therapist performs joint mobilization for therapeutic purposes and can employ any number of movement variations depending on the purpose for applying mobilization. These movements can be fast or slow, vigorous or gentle, or have a broad or narrow sweep.

It is generally beneficial to warm up a joint prior to vigorous use. Mobilization movements can assist in preparing a joint for activity by warming the joint through enhanced circulation and by gently stretching the surrounding musculature.

Rocking is a simple type of joint mobilization. Rocking is performed by moving a body part rhythmically from side to side or back and forth. Rocking may be accompanied by compression, as in rocking compression, or by jostling, when muscles are shaken loosely back and forth (see Figure 3.3).

Mobilization is also beneficial in remediation of athletic injuries. It can assist in reducing apprehension and voluntary splinting associated with pain, thereby reducing circulatory-retained metabolites and muscle-tissue ischemia. Such therapy results in early functional mobility, which is essential to quick recovery. Mobilization for remediation must be performed within the comfort zone. The athlete should not feel pain from the movement. (See "Remedial Massage" on page 49).

Stretching

The healthy flexible body can move freely and easily through its natural ROM without discomfort and restrictions in the joints and surrounding tissues. Physical and psychological stress or trauma can result in restricted flexibility. Inflexibility reduces the athletic potential and increases the risk of injury. It is no wonder that flexibility training is considered one of the most important aspects of athletic conditioning.

Stretching has long been a key element in programs for improving flexibility. It is used in sports massage, usually following treatment, to enhance the flexibility gained by the actual manipulation of the tissues involved in the restriction.

Stretching has gone through several changes in philosophy in the course of its long history. The earliest stretches were ballistic, or bouncing, stretches followed by static stretches that hold the stretch for an extended period of time. The most recent version of stretching, proprioceptive neuromuscular facilitation (PNF), alternately contracts and stretches the muscle.

Ballistic stretching has fallen from use in all but the most controlled situations, as it is believed to place the athlete at risk of an overstretch injury. Static stretching is still considered effective for enhancing flexibility and is the most popular method of stretching. *Stretching* by Anderson (1980) and *Sport Stretch* by Alter (1990) are excellent resources for static stretching techniques and are especially good for athletes; they include stretching routines for various sports. PNF was recently hailed as the best stretching method; however, new studies have raised questions about earlier studies and show little evidence that PNF is better than static stretching. PNF is a complex system of promoting a desired muscular response, and physical therapists use it for purposes other than stretching. Therefore, we include here a brief description of the three PNF techniques commonly used in sports massage for the purposes of increasing flexibility.

Contract/Relax

The athlete contracts and then relaxes a muscle or muscle group. The intentional contracting of a muscle can facilitate a greater subsequent relaxation of that muscle. This technique relaxes muscles in a chronic hypertonic condition brought on by either mental or emotional stress or repetitive use.

For example, an athlete who is feeling the pressures of the upcoming meet can experience hypertonic levator scapulae muscles. In addition to therapy, the coach can instruct the athlete to perform simple contract/relax techniques throughout the day. By raising his or her shoulders toward the ears, the athlete will be contracting the levator scapulae. After a firm contraction the athlete simply lets go of the tension, letting the shoulders relax and drop down. Repeating this several times in a row reduces the hypertonic condition; performing these sets several times each day can result in normalized tissue and thus enhance athletic performance.

Contract/Relax/Stretch

The athlete contracts and then relaxes a muscle or muscle group. The therapist applies a stretch to the muscle immediately following the relaxation of that muscle. For example, the therapist will offer resistance to the athlete's hamstring muscle group and instruct the athlete to contract the hamstrings against that resistance. When the athlete discontinues the contraction and relaxes the hamstrings, the therapist immediately applies a stretch to the hamstrings.

This technique takes advantage of the greater relaxation to produce a stretch. It enhances the muscle elongation potential and thus the ROM of any articulation where muscle tightness causes restriction.

Contract/Relax/Stretch Using Reciprocal Inhibition

The athlete contracts and then relaxes a muscle or muscle group. The therapist applies a stretch to the antagonist muscle immediately following the relaxation of the agonist muscle. For example, the therapist will offer resistance to the athlete's quadriceps muscle group and instruct the athlete to contract the quadriceps against that resistance. When the athlete discontinues the contraction and relaxes the quadriceps, the therapist immediately applies a stretch to the hamstrings.

This method utilizes the natural response of reciprocal inhibition to produce a greater stretch. Reciprocal inhibition is the component of the neuromuscular mechanism that determines that in order for movement to occur during contraction of the agonist muscle, the antagonist muscle must relax. We utilize that relaxation of the antagonist muscle as an opportunity to stretch it more effectively. This technique is most beneficial whenever the therapist does not want the muscle needing to be stretched to contract, such as when reducing a muscle cramp.

Positional Release

One of the most useful new techniques in sports massage was developed by a chiropractor named Lawrence Jones. It is called *strain-counterstrain*, or in its generic form, *positional release*. It is an effective and noninvasive method to ease acute tension or spasm.

In positional release, a "tender point" is located near an area of muscle tension. A tender point is a small area that can be found by palpation with the thumb or fingertip and that when pressed is more tender than the surrounding area. This point is used to find the correct joint position for helping the tense muscle to relax.

Positional release is simple in concept and includes four steps (Chaitow, 1988, pp. 247-248):

1. Find the tender point in a muscle.

2. Hold the tender point while moving the joint to a position in which pain is diminished.

3. Hold the position for 90 seconds.

4. Return the area to its neutral resting position.

The positional release of a tight latissimus dorsi is described using the four steps in Figure 2.32, a through d. Use the four steps of positional release on a tense muscle. Positional release is especially useful because it is gentle and does not cause the more intense discomfort associated with some deep-muscle techniques, such as deep-digital pressure on trigger points. Positional release may be used to address chronic tension as well as acute situations.

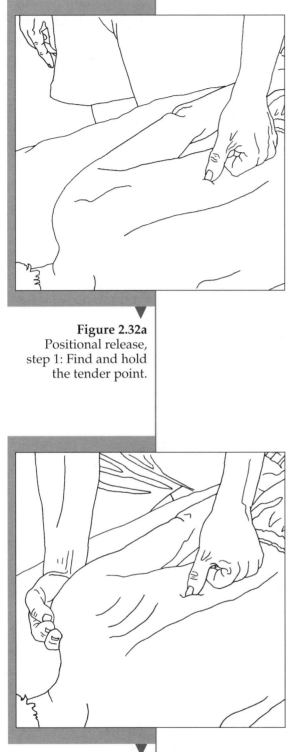

Figure 2.32a
Positional release,
step 1: Find and hold
the tender point.

Figure 2.32b
Positional release,
step 2: Move the
associated joint to
the position of
diminished pain.

Figure 2.32c
Positional release,
step 3: Hold the tender
point and the joint in
the position of dimin-
ished pain for 90
seconds.

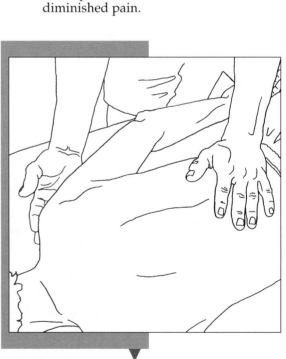

Figure 2.32d
Positional release,
step 4: Return the area
to its neutral resting
position.

PALPATION

Perhaps the most basic and crucial skill in giving sports massage is palpation. At its simplest level, palpation is the ability to locate with the hands specific structures such as bony landmarks, as well as individual muscles, their transition to tendon, and finally their points of attachment. This ability adds the quality of specificity to the session. For example, Figure 2.33 shows palpation of the biceps brachii at the point of attachment at the shoulder.

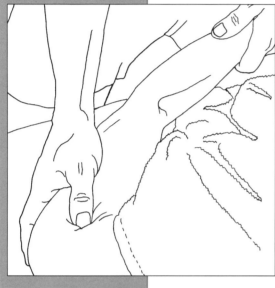

During passive joint mobilization and stretching, information about the condition of a joint can be surmised through certain qualities of the movements (e.g., crepitations, drag, or "end feel"). Palpatory information may help locate the source of interference with normal ROM.

In addition, massage specialists learn to recognize the texture of the tissues, their degree of tension, and the difference between firm and tense muscle. Hypertonic muscle is hard and ropelike; healthy muscle tissue is firm yet elastic and broad or flat, not round. Massage specialists can also sense where tissues are adhering; identify conditions such as scarring, edema, and fibrosis; and locate specific points of tension such as trigger points.

More importantly, it is possible to detect changes in the tissues and movement qualities during a session and from one session to the next. This provides important feedback concerning the effectiveness of specific techniques and approaches.

Figure 2.33
Palpation of the biceps brachii.

In this chapter, we have described the basic techniques of sports massage, including palpatory skills, common hand positions, and traditional and contemporary massage movements. These basic manual techniques are combined and applied in various situations and for a variety of purposes; ultimately, however, they all aim to enhance performance. The techniques described are not intended to represent the full spectrum of massage skills, but rather to represent those most often used in the sport setting.

The next two chapters describe how to use these basic techniques for recovery and remediation and during or between competitive events.

CHAPTER 3

RESTORATIVE MASSAGE

Sport activity can be physically, psychologically, and emotionally demanding for athletes of all ages and skill levels. Participation in sports repeatedly places the player at risk of injury, and the training and practice required to become skillful often result in overuse conditions. Even successful practice sessions leave the athlete tired, drained of energy, and physiologically depleted.

Recovering from such bouts of activity and restoring the athlete to a preinjury level of physical and psychological competitive fitness are the goals of *restorative massage*. Taken a step further is the hope of exceeding the previous level of fitness to avoid future injury.

Restorative massage has three major applications based on the extent of the condition being treated.

- *Recovery massage* for the uninjured athlete needing recovery from a strenuous workout or competition

- *Remedial massage* for minor to moderate injuries

- *Rehabilitation massage* for severe injury or following surgical intervention

This chapter explains how to use massage to restore athletes to optimal condition from various levels of debility and gives specific examples of sports massage protocol for several common injuries.

RECOVERY MASSAGE

Sports massage given after a strenuous workout or competition can enhance the athlete's physiological and psychological recovery from the stress of that activity. It augments the body's own healing and recovery processes and helps the athlete to maintain a state of dynamic equilibrium during the seasons of training and competition or as part of an ongoing fitness program.

Sports massage facilitates recovery by increasing circulation, which promotes better cell nutrition and removal of waste products, by relaxing tight muscles, and by inducing general mind–body relaxation.

The duration of the treatment for recovery depends on its proximity to competition. Soon after competition the duration is shorter, usually about 30 minutes. Several hours after competition or the following day, a recovery session may last an hour. The techniques commonly used for recovery are deep sliding movements (with oil), kneading, compression (without oil), positional release, skin rolling, joint mobilization, and stretching. The tempo is relaxing and the techniques are applied to the entire body with specific attention to the muscle groups most stressed during physical activity. Deep breathing and other relaxation techniques are appropriate adjuncts to recovery massage. The addition of a whirlpool, sauna, steam, or a hot shower also augments the recovery massage.

General guidelines for recovery sports massage suggest that the massage should

- aim to improve circulation and promote muscular and general relaxation;
- last from 30 minutes to 1 hour;
- include techniques used for recovery such as sliding movements, kneading, compression, positional release, skin rolling, joint mobilizations, and stretching;
- spend more time on areas most stressed in recent activity; and
- use adjunct methods such as deep breathing and other relaxation techniques, including a whirlpool, sauna, steam, or hot shower.

While the need for a quick recovery and restoration to normalcy is indisputable (the quicker the better for competitive athletes), this normal recovery process is not considered pathophysiologic and therefore is not of particular interest to the physical therapist or athletic trainer. Because massage can enhance and hasten recovery, it is worth having a sports massage specialist apply it. However, recovery massage is a simple style of massage, and anyone who takes the time to learn the necessary techniques can safely apply it. Coaches, athletic trainers, teammates, and even family members can all assist athletes by giving recovery massage.

Massage at the YMCA

By 1915, when R. Tait McKenzie described the YMCA's program of exercise, the rubdown had become an established part of the routine. According to McKenzie, workouts at the YMCA included a mixture of Swedish and German gymnastics and games, "ending with a bath and a rub down" (p. 170).

As health service at the Y grew through the years, massage continued to be an important part of it. The emphasis was on helping people stay healthy, what would be called a fitness or wellness approach today. Two hundred seventy-four YMCAs in the United States were operating health service sections by 1943.

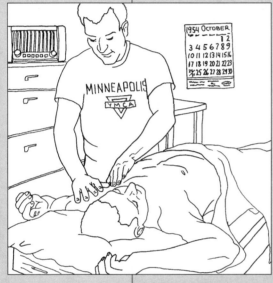

The Dayton Association in Ohio established a School of Health Service and Massage in 1937 to train practitioners, called operators or technicians, for the YMCA. In the early 1940s its summer refresher clinic for older, more experienced masseurs included the care and prevention of athletic injuries and corrective and rehabilitation work.

In 1942 the YMCA formed a Health Service Operators Society to promote health services within the Ys and "to combat the abuses of commercial bath houses and the unethical conduct of 'cure-all' agents in the health field" (Williams, 1943, p. 30). Health service operators, also called masseurs, received college credit through George Williams College in Chicago for a national clinic sponsored by the Health Service Operators Society in 1947 (Johnson, n.d., p. 313). This professional society was active through the 1950s.

During these years massage operators at the Y worked with healthy people to promote fitness and enhance physical activity. The scope of their practice and methods was described by Frierwood in 1953:

> The technician uses massage, baths (shower, steam, electricity cabinet), ultraviolet irradiation (artificial and natural sunlight), infrared (heat), instruction in relaxation and in some cases directed exercise. The adult members secure a relief from tensions, gain a sense of well-being, give attention to personal fitness and develop habits designed to build and maintain optimum health and physical efficiency throughout the lifespan. (p. 21)

Although the YMCA training programs for massage specialists disappeared by the 1960s, massage continues to be offered as a health service, continuing a tradition of over 80 years.

SAMPLE RECOVERY MASSAGE WITHOUT OIL

Recovery sports massage may be given without using oil or other lubricants. The athlete receiving the massage may wear shorts and a T-shirt or a warm-up suit, the clothing satisfying issues of modesty.

Several massage techniques that facilitate recovery are performed easily and effectively through clothing, including compression, rocking, jostling, shaking, kneading, percussion, friction, vibration, skin rolling, broadening, digital compression, and joint mobilizations and stretching. Apply these techniques sequentially to each part of the body: First warm up each part, follow with more specific work, and end with nonspecific connecting and finishing techniques.

Prone Position

The athlete lies facedown. Place a bolster or rolled towel under the ankles for support or let the feet hang off the end of the table.

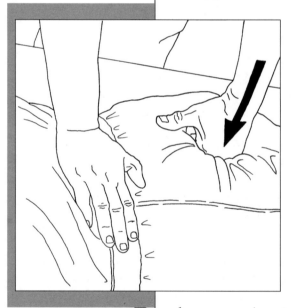

Figure 3.1
Compression on the buttocks using a fist.

Legs

Begin warming up the entire left leg and hip, using rocking compression and jostling. Follow with more specific massage on each part in order, starting with the buttocks, upper leg, lower leg, and finishing with the feet.

Compression and kneading are effective on the large muscles of the buttocks. Figure 3.1 shows compression on the buttocks using a fist. Use broadening, jostling, and kneading on the upper leg and then the lower leg. Hold the anterior ankle while you flex the lower leg, bringing the heel of the foot toward the buttocks for a gentle stretch of the quadriceps. With the lower leg flexed to a 90-degree angle, perform some joint mobilizations of the ankle. Hold the foot at a comfortable angle and use your fist to apply compressions to the bottom of the foot.

Finish with a few light palmar sliding movements, light hacking, or slapping over the clothing from the foot to the buttocks to reconnect the leg and create a feeling of wholeness. Repeat on the right side.

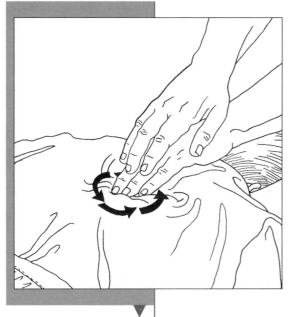

Figure 3.2
Circular friction on
the erector spinae.

Back

Use compression and rocking compression to warm up the back. Follow with kneading the shoulders and use circular friction of the erector muscles along the spine (see Figure 3.2). Perform skin rolling to the entire back, especially along the spine and over the scapulae. Finish with light sliding movements, cupping, or hacking over the back from the shoulders to the hips. Don't forget the sides.

Supine Position

The athlete lies faceup. Place a bolster under the knees to take pressure off the lower back. A small towel may be used as a neck roll for support.

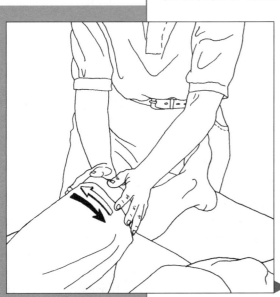

Legs

Warm up the front of the left leg, using compression and rocking compression. Begin specific work on the upper leg, applying broadening, kneading, and jostling. Add friction around the knees. Apply compression along the tibialis anterior, pressing away from the tibia. Then add friction around the ankle. Apply digital compression to the dorsal foot and mobilize the foot bones. Finish with light palmar sliding movements from the ankle to the hip, and then jostle the muscles of the leg while moving your hands from the hip to the foot (see Figure 3.3). Repeat on the right side.

 Figure 3.3 Jostling the leg from side to side.

Chest

Use compression with the fist to warm up the pectorals. Follow with circular friction. Stretch the arms overhead. Finish with light tapping over the chest. Be sure to avoid touching breast tissue in women.

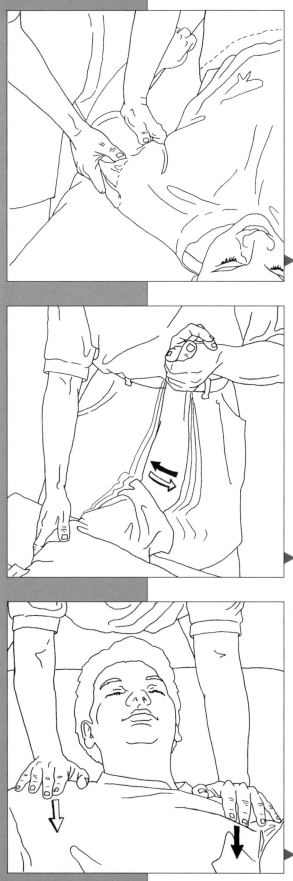

Arm and Shoulder

Gently squeeze the left arm in your two hands, moving along from shoulder to wrist as shown in Figure 3.4. Repeat twice to warm the area. Continue with more specific work in sequence, from the upper arm to the lower arm, wrist, and then the hand.

Perform compression, kneading, and broadening on the shoulder and upper arm. Use the same techniques on the lower arm, varying your hand position to effectively address the smaller size.

▶ **Figure 3.4**   Squeezing and broadening the muscles of the arm using two hands.

Use friction with the thumbs around the wrist. Mobilize all of the joints of the hand. Perform thumb slides on the palm of the hand.

To mobilize and relax the whole arm, grasp the hand and bend the arm to a 90-degree angle, lift the upper arm slightly off the table, and then wag the arm from side to side, gently moving the wrist, elbow, and shoulder (see Figure 3.5). Finish with light sliding movements from the shoulder to the hand.

▶ **Figure 3.5**   Mobilizing the arm using wagging movements.

Neck and Head

Apply light friction to the back and sides of the neck, using multiple-digit placement. The joints of the neck will mobilize as you push up on the neck muscles. Apply digital compression to the occipital ridge.

Then add light friction to the sides and top of the head. Finish with light sliding movements from the shoulder to the head along both sides. To end the session, stand at the head and mobilize each shoulder by pressing forward with a cat-like movement, alternating sides as shown in Figure 3.6. Hold the shoulders lightly for a few seconds before breaking contact.

▶ **Figure 3.6**   Mobilizing the shoulders using alternating pressing toward the feet.

REMEDIAL MASSAGE

Injuries and debilitating conditions occur with unfortunate regularity in both amateur and professional athletes. Even minor conditions can hamper athletic performance and can lead to more serious injury if left unchecked. Massage therapy that is intended to resolve or assist the athlete with such conditions is called *remedial massage*. The main goal of remedial massage is to restore the athlete to a preinjury level of physical and psychological fitness, and perhaps even exceed the previous level of fitness to avoid future injuries. Remedial massage is specific in its approach and is results oriented. Practitioners require additional training, knowledge, and skills to give safe and effective treatments; remedial massage should not be attempted by unqualified persons.

Remedial massage is applied to conditions such as muscle tension, sprains, strains, and tendinitis and in the treatment of specific debilitating pathologies such as shin splints or tennis elbow. When included in the overall treatment protocol, remedial massage often offers athletes a faster, more complete recovery from such injuries.

This approach to massage also investigates the biomechanical factors arising from or causing the condition. The primary objective of remedial massage is to reduce or eliminate the complaint, which is typically pain or dysfunction. After the pain or symptoms have been addressed, the therapist may investigate methods to prevent recurrence of the complaint, to maintain symptomatic relief, or if the condition is resolved, to educate the athlete on the benefits of wellness massage.

In the sport environment there are many conditions that do not require surgical intervention. Standard medical advice for nonsurgical conditions ranges from simply "Do nothing, it will go away on its own" to recommendations for ice and anti-inflammatories and referral to physical therapy. Referral to a sports massage therapist has become increasingly popular because massage is now recognized as one of the most significant mechanisms for assisting conditions that fall somewhere between doing nothing and surgical intervention. The do-nothing approach is no longer acceptable to educated athletes. Sports massage can help them achieve faster, more complete recovery than simple rest. Massage treatment of minor injuries also reduces the risk of injury recurrence, improves the potential for early mobilization, and improves the mental attitude of injured athletes by getting them back to practice before they lose their conditioning.

Because the do-nothing approach is so widespread, and because the sports massage therapist has direct access to the public, athletes with minor problems are increasingly seeking out sports massage therapists as the *first* source for consultation.

Remedial massage treatments, due to their specific goals, can last from 5 to 15 minutes at the injury site. Because a therapist may need to work with the surrounding tissues as well, a treatment may be extended to 30 minutes. The tempo depends on the specific goals of each treatment. Treatments are usually given two to three times per week depending on the condition. The frequency of visits decreases as the athlete returns to normal activity.

Remedial Massage Applications

The following sections describe some of the most common remedial applications in sports massage.

Muscle Tension and Inflexibility

Although range of motion (ROM) limitations typically determine the amount of flexibility in a muscle or muscle group, this measurement is not always an accurate indicator. A joint that is suffering a structural problem, such as a bone spur or arthritis, may exhibit restriction in ROM while the surrounding musculature may be flexible, or pliable. In an opposite scenario, a gymnast may be hypermobile in joint ROM and have tight, nonpliable muscles. The sports massage therapist will use palpation to determine muscle flexibility. When muscle tension limits joint ROM, massage therapy is very effective in improving ROM (or flexibility).

There are many causes of muscle inflexibility:

- Any period of immobility will shorten the stretch reflex of the muscle–tendon component.

- Scar tissue is less flexible than muscle tissue and excessive amounts, or any amount in the wrong place, may result in lack of flexibility.

- Edema (any swelling in the tissue) will reduce flexibility. The pressure of excessive fluids within the edemic area irritates the nerve endings.

- Fascial thickening is the body's response to stress in either chronic or acute situations. Fascia that is thickened is less pliable and will reduce flexibility in the involved muscle.

- Voluntary and involuntary muscle splinting due to pain causes inflexibility.

- Chronic muscle tension results in muscle contraction and muscle shortening, eventually leading to fascial thickening and muscle inflexibility.

- Apprehension and emotional stress can result in muscle tension and an unconscious tightening of muscles.

Massage therapy protocol for muscle inflexibility centers around determining the cause of the inflexibility and utilizing techniques to counteract such causes. It is important to note the difference between chronic and acute muscle tension because the massage treatment for each is different.

Chronic muscle tension progresses slowly. It is caused by poor posture, excessive repetition of a particular movement (repetitive use syndrome), consistent inefficient biomechanical movement patterns, and unconscious holding of tension or emotional stress. The physiology will contain components of fascial thickening, trigger points, adhesions, eschemia, and possibly crepitation. In some cases of chronic muscle tension the complaint centers around a burning neuralgia or myositis; in others the result is a sensation of dulling the sensitivity in the area often referred to as "armoring." In either case there is significant pain on palpation. Other symptoms include fatigue and loss of muscle flexibility and power. These symptoms combine to set up the pain-spasm-pain cycle and perpetuate the chronic nature of the condition.

Massage techniques that increase circulation, encourage fascial lengthening, and reduce adhesions and trigger points address chronic muscle conditions. Working with the concept of the *optimal therapy zone* during the session also provides significant and quick results. Massage techniques might include sliding movements, deep-transverse friction, compression, myofasical release, positional release, deep-digital pressure, jostling, and PNF.

It is best to approach *acute muscle tension* from a different perspective. The muscle tension occurs suddenly either from recent overuse (delayed onset soreness) or emotional tension (most often in the form of performance anxiety). Any deep massage would only aggravate the tissue, and probably the athlete as well. Juhan (1987) suggests that force cannot be used to make a muscle relax and lengthen and that the quality of movement must be slow and nonthreatening to effect relaxation. He maintains that physical and emotional pleasure are essential in "interrupting self-perpetuating cycles of excess tension," and that pain and discomfort are counterproductive because they trigger the body's defense systems (p. 206). This view echoes Galen's advice that in "rubbing" after exercise the "hard kinds" should be avoided, and that movements should be quick and soft "to carry off the excretions and soften the tense parts" (Johnson 1866, p. 25). This runs counter to the stereotypical picture of the big, bruising masseur or masseuse pummeling muscles into submission while the client screams in pain.

Massage techniques that increase circulation, reduce local nerve excitability, evoke a neuromuscular relaxation reflex, and produce overall relaxation are effective in reducing acute muscle tension. Massage techniques might include sliding strokes, vibration, compression, jostling, joint mobilization, and PNF.

In addition to performing appropriate massage therapy techniques, the therapist should suggest ways to reduce the causative factors of chronic or acute muscle tension and teach the use of self-massage and stretching for more frequent treatment of overused muscles. Coaches may help correct biomechanical movement patterns, improper use of equipment, or use of the incorrect equipment. Athletes may also learn general relaxation techniques such as progressive relaxation, autogenic suggestion, and deep breathing.

Muscle Soreness

Muscle soreness is familiar to all athletes—from weekend warriors to elite competitors. Some distinguish what they call "acute muscle pain" from "delayed onset soreness." Acute muscle pain is thought to be related to muscle ischemia brought on by intense exercise of short duration, which decreases when the ischemia is removed. Delayed muscle soreness, on the other hand, "increases for 2 to 3 days following strenuous exercise, usually peaks in intensity 24 to 48 hours post exercise, and thereafter slowly diminishes disappearing at 5 to 7 days after exercise" (Yackzan, Adams, & Francis, 1984, p. 159). Three theories are proposed to explain delayed muscle soreness: tonic muscle spasm, torn tissue (microtears), and connective tissue damage.

Two other theories trace postexercise muscle soreness to retention of metabolites (by-products of muscle activity) and low-level edema. These conditions may irritate nervous tissue and cause pain in the area. Any or all of the five conditions listed above may result in the pain or various degrees of soreness after exercise.

Massage is an excellent treatment for muscle soreness of all kinds because one of its primary effects is to increase circulation of blood and lymph. Increased blood and lymph flow to an area brings better cell nutrition, carries away metabolites, reduces edema, and promotes healing of damaged tissues.

The best techniques for increased circulation are sliding movements, kneading, and compression. The pressure used in applying these techniques should be carefully monitored. Very sore areas should receive light pressure; increase pressure as the soreness diminishes.

Stretching before and after exercise is also reported to help reduce muscular soreness.

Trigger Points

Trigger points undoubtedly account for much of the myofascial pain and dysfunction that athletes in heavy training experience. According to Travell and Simons (1983), acute overload, overwork fatigue, direct trauma, and chilling activate trigger points, and they frequently develop in muscles subject to excessive repetitive or sustained contractions (p. 14).

Trigger points are defined as

a focus of hyperirritability in a tissue that, when compressed, is locally tender and, if sufficiently hypersensitive, gives rise to referred pain and tenderness, and sometimes to referred autonomic phenomena and distortion of proprioception. (Travell & Simons, 1983, p. 4)

Signs of trigger points may include dull, aching, or deep referred pain; variable irritability over time; stiffness and weakness in the involved muscle; restricted range of motion; pain on contraction; and pain on stretching. Pain will often be experienced out of proportion to the pressure applied directly to the area and felt either in the immediate area or remote from the point (Travell & Simons, 1983, pp. 13-17).

Trigger points may be felt during palpation as a taut band or spot of tissue distinguishable from surrounding tissue. They are best relieved by direct digital pressure. Figure 3.7 shows the application of direct digital pressure to a trigger point in the pectoralis minor, followed by a stretch of that muscle (Figure 3.8). Stretching helps to reeducate the muscle as to its increased length after the treatment. Deep sliding movements with the thumb, kneading, pincement, and vibration supplement direct pressure to trigger points. These other massage techniques are used to warm up the area, aid in the release of the trigger point, and help the tissue recover from the effects of ischemia that accompanies trigger points. In some instances, positional release is also effective with trigger points.

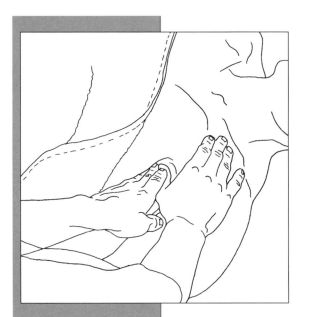

Figure 3.7
Digital pressure to a
trigger point in the
pectoralis minor.

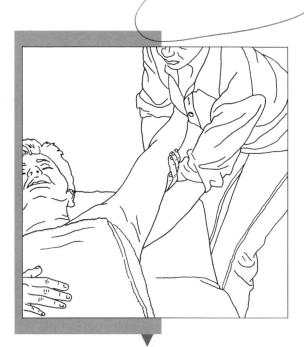

Figure 3.8
Stretching the
pectoralis minor.

Edema

Edema is simply "the abnormal accumulation of fluid in interstitial spaces of tissues" (Anderson & Anderson, 1990, p. 303). It may result in noticeable and palpable swelling of tissues, soreness or pain, and restricted movement around joints.

We expect edema to be present in most injuries, but it may also accompany delayed muscle soreness, minor strains, sprains, tendinitis, and hyperemia after strenuous exercise.

Edema may be relieved with long, sliding massage movements in a distal to proximal direction. Pressure should be light directly over the edema and continue with deeper pressure proximal to the area.

Contraindications for massage of edema should be carefully noted; they include acute inflammation, heart disease, and kidney disease. Although generally contraindicated under these conditions, massage may be received under certain circumstances with the direct supervision of a physician (Tappan, 1988, pp. 28-30).

Tendinitis

Tendon inflammation (*tendinitis*) is a common condition among athletes and may be the result of poor biomechanics, repetitive motion, irritation, or a sudden increase in workload. Once tendinitis sets in, it causes pain and interferes with performance.

One of the benefits of regular maintenance massage is that the therapist can detect subclinical tendinitis during a massage session. *Subclinical* refers to a condition that does not present overt symptoms. Subclinical tendinitis is painful under the pressure of massage, but the athlete will

Tennis Elbow

Tennis elbow is a common tendinitis complaint. Most cases involve the wrist extensor muscles, which attach to the lateral epicondyle of the humerus; thus it is often referred to as lateral epicondylitis. Massage for tennis elbow includes deep-transverse friction of the tendons near the point of attachment and kneading to relieve chronic tension of the associated muscles.

Pain in the elbow can arise from numerous conditions that must be considered and evaluated prior to treatment. The elbow should not be catching or locking, there should be no neurological symptoms, and there should be no significant restriction of passive range of motion.

The onset of tennis elbow is usually gradual, brought on by overuse rather than some sudden trauma. As with any strain or tendinitis condition, there will be pain at a specific site (point tenderness at the lateral epicondyle of the humerus); this pain may be elicited on active, resistive muscle testing. Swelling, tightness, and discomfort along the involved muscle are also possible.

Treatment for tennis elbow begins with ice therapy and anti-inflammatory drugs to address the inflammation and edema. Modification of activity is important but does not mean bed rest. The tennis player should use the next few days to concentrate training on footwork and aerobic conditioning while reducing the use of the arm.

Massage therapy begins with a warm-up of the entire upper extremity and includes long sliding movements from wrist to shoulder, gentle kneading to both the anterior and posterior musculature, and compression. As the tissue becomes warm and pliable the amount of pressure may be increased and the massage techniques change from general to specific.

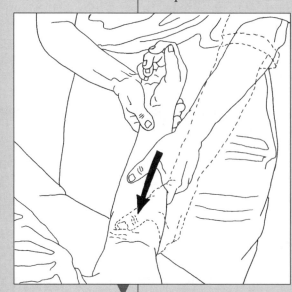

Figure A

A unique application of the sliding movement, called "draining," is used on the forearm (see Figure A). The athlete is in supine position with his or her elbow flexed to 90 degrees. The athlete's upper arm is resting on the table while you hold the forearm in a vertical position. Encourage the athlete to relax the forearm musculature. While holding the athlete's arm up with one hand, use your other hand to perform a deep sliding movement from the wrist to the elbow. The feel of the technique is of draining all the fluid from the forearm toward the elbow. Repeat the sliding motion all the way around the forearm. This movement may elicit pain in tight muscles and should be performed with care; use an even, steady pace.

Place the elbow into extension, resting the entire arm on the table with the forearm pronated, and continue to use the thumb on the extensor muscles with slow, sliding movements. The movement should be from the wrist to just above the elbow, and the area will be tender as you pass over the tendons at the elbow. This is a good time to add active movement to the sliding technique. You can accomplish this by asking the athlete to flex and extend the wrist as you perform the sliding movement. The result will be amplified as the muscle contracts and relaxes. The movement should again be done at a slow and steady pace. You may also switch from sliding to digital pressure with active movement; place your thumb on a tight place in the muscle and have the athlete extend and then relax the wrist, move to another location, and repeat. This is very effective near to and at the tendon site.

The most effective massage technique for tennis elbow is deep-transverse friction (see pages 32-33). When performing friction as a remedial technique, it is important to combine the treatment with ice massage. Apply about 8 minutes of ice massage to the lateral elbow prior to friction; then during the treatment you can periodically interrupt the friction with a minute of ice massage. This will help reduce the discomfort level for the athlete and allow a more effective treatment as well as reduce the inflammation response.

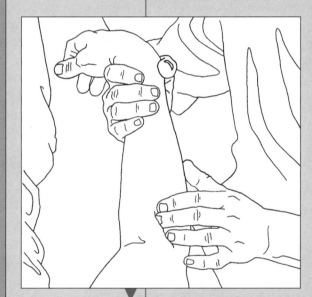

Figure B

To best perform friction to the extensor tendons, with the athlete supine, place the upper extremity in an internally rotated position and abducted approximately 45 degrees (see Figure B). Appy deep-transverse friction on and around the extensor muscle attachments at the lateral epicondyle of the humerus. Be sure to either support the elbow with your hand or have it placed on the table. This position ensures that the tendon is in proper position for the frictioning, thus greatly improving the results of the treatment.

The frictioning is always painful on tendinitis and should be followed by comforting and soothing sliding movements. Also it is best to end the session with one more ice treatment and have the athlete perform about 60 seconds of active movement at the wrist. This entire session could be completed in 15 to 30 minutes.

report being previously unaware that any problem was present. The common joke is, "My elbow was fine until you pressed on it!" In reality, the tendon was not "fine" and if left alone would likely develop into a full tendinitis condition with pain and diminished function. If subclinical tendinitis is detected in the course of a massage session, the athlete, the coach, and the athletic trainer can begin a comprehensive treatment approach. Quick action can prevent a more serious problem and avert any detrimental effect on performance.

The standard treatment for subclinical tendinitis and for cases of tendinitis exhibiting moderate symptoms is the same: cryotherapy (including ice massage), anti-inflammatories, deep-transverse friction massage, modification of activity, and correction of improper biomechanics. It is essential to emphasize frequent use of ice and anti-inflammatories when the treatment protocol includes deep-transverse friction massage. Without proper use of ice and nonsteroidal anti-inflammatory drugs (NSAIDs), deep-transverse friction massage would further irritate the tissue. Additionally, general relaxing massage of the tendon's associated muscle will reduce the irritation of the tendon and provide a more effective environment for healing.

In severe cases of tendinitis deep-transverse friction massage may be contraindicated until the condition has improved. Massage to reduce spasm and tension in the associated muscle is beneficial during this early stage, and deep-transverse friction massage may be added to the treatment session once inflammation has subsided.

Tenosynovitis

Tenosynovitis is inflammation of the thin synovial lining of the sheath covering a tendon and may be the result of mechanical irritation or bacterial infection. Symptoms in the acute phase include sudden crepitus and edema, and in the chronic phase, local thickening. A physician must determine the causative factor and treatment protocol.

Massage therapy for tenosynovitis is the same as therapy for tendinitis only more care is given to have the tendon on stretch during the application of deep-transverse friction. Cyriax and Cyriax (1993, p. 19) explain that "it appears that the manual rolling of the tendon sheath to and fro against the tendon serves to smooth off the roughened surfaces." If mechanical cause is determined, measures to eliminate or reduce those causative factors must be explored with the coach or athletic trainer.

Strains

A *strain* is the damage of some part of the muscle, fascia, or tendon brought on by overuse (chronic strain) or overstress (acute strain). The acute strain is usually related to sudden changes of tension in the muscle created by violent stretch or rapid contraction. Sudden bursts of power, such as charging to the net in tennis or sprinting in track, or sudden stretching, such as landing a dismount with hyperextended knees in gymnastics, are some examples of the kinds of activity that cause strains. A muscle may also strain as a result of decelerating a rapid movement, such as pitching a baseball.

A *Grade 1 strain* is characterized by low-grade inflammation, edema, and mild discomfort in use. There may be no apparent loss of ROM or strength, and there will be no palpable defect in the tissues. However, partial tearing or microtears may be present and spasm or edema may cause pain.

Treatment consists of ice and massage. Begin with light sliding massage movements to improve circulation and reduce edema. Next apply massage with moderate pressure to the surrounding muscle to reduce muscle spasm. As pain subsides, more vigorous massage and massage to the specific injury site will return the injured muscle–tendon area to optimal function.

For example, massage a mildly strained quadriceps with a combination of sliding, vibration, and kneading. Keep the pressure and pace of the movements lighter and slower at first and increase them as the pain subsides either during one session or over a series of spaced sessions.

A *Grade 2 strain* has definite inflammation and edema with possible hemorrhaging. The athlete will experience severe discomfort with use, voluntary or involuntary muscle splinting, and discernible loss in ROM and strength. There will be a palpable lesion in the muscle or tendon.

Treatment requires ice and modification of activity (rest). Due to the severity of the injury, massage directly over the injured site is contraindicated. However, massage to the muscles proximal to the injured area may help reduce the edema. Care must be taken to work well within the comfort zone.

Several days postinjury, more vigorous massage may be applied around, but not directly on, the injury site to assist in the removal of debris caused by hemorrhage. Gentle sliding movements may be applied directly over the injury site to help reduce edema, taking care to stay in the athlete's comfort zone.

Once the area has had significant reduction of swelling and the hemorrhage begins to dissipate, apply moderate massage to the entire length of the muscle. If it can be accomplished with little discomfort, more vigorous techniques may be added. During the final stages of healing, apply deep-transverse friction directly to the injury site to address adhesions and scarring.

Massage therapy is very effective at speeding recovery from Grade 2 strains. However, it is important to note that massage applied inappropriately can cause further trauma to the injured tissues. If the injury is severe or if you question the appropriateness of treatment, it is important that you refer the injured athlete to a sports medicine physician for diagnosis. Only massage therapists with specialized skills and training for treating sport injuries and athletic trainers and physical therapists who are trained in massage should attempt to treat a Grade 2 muscle strain with massage therapy.

A *Grade 3 strain* is characterized by severe inflammation, edema with discoloration, and severely impaired function of the affected muscle. There will be a definite palpable lesion, possibly accompanied by muscle "bunching." Always refer suspected Grade 3 strains to a physician for diagnosis. Treatment may include surgical intervention. In the absence of surgery and with referral by a physician, massage may be performed as in a Grade 2 strain. Time lines for healing should be extended appropriately, and complete rest should be encouraged.

Sprains

As strains are to muscle, sprains are to ligaments. A *sprain* most often follows a sudden forced stretch of a joint beyond its normal ROM, which results in damage to the joint's ligaments and other stabilizing structures. Sprains range from those exhibiting no significant loss of function (Grade 1) to those where complete rupture and loss of function occur

(Grade 3). Sprains can be a serious matter and may require surgical intervention. In addition, what may appear to be a sprain may in fact be a fracture; therefore, it is best to refer most sprains to a physician for diagnosis.

In early stages of healing of any sprain use rest, ice, compression, and elevation (RICE) to address inflammation and edema. Mobilizations without pain, done in the early stages and continued throughout the healing process, help keep joints supple and speed the return to normal ROM. Sliding massage movements applied to the tissues around, but not on, the injured part can also be done in the early stages to help reduce edema and improve circulation.

Muscles surrounding the affected joint frequently become tense from the trauma itself and the accompanying pain. In addition, muscles in other areas may become tense from either protective holding or modified movement patterns (e.g., limping). Such tension can cause additional pain and debilitating conditions. Massage, as described earlier in this section, can help relieve this type of muscle tension and spasm.

After the acute phase when the injury is healed, deep-transverse friction applied directly to the injury site can assist in the formation of a functional scar (see Figure 3.9). This type of treatment should be done carefully and only by those trained to do so. The healing ligament will often attach itself to the bone at a site where the ligament is designed to slide over the surface of the bone. This adhesion can produce chronic pain cycles for athletes as they injure, heal, and reinjure this ligament due to its dysfunctional condition. The use of deep-transverse friction massage will eliminate this adhesion and restore the ligament to a functional condition.

Strengthening exercises should be performed on the healed sprain. These exercises are intended not only to restore the muscle to its preinjury condition but also to add dynamic stability through muscle strength and compensate for any possible loss of static stability from ligament weakness.

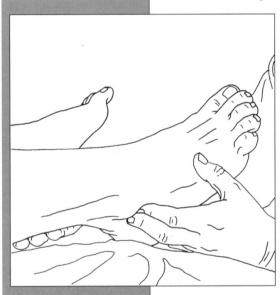

Figure 3.9 Deep-transverse friction to the ankle.

Stress

Moderate stress can be stimulating and invigorating. However, the pressures of training and competition added to the stress from school or work, family and friends, and other life situations may result in nearly debilitating levels of stress. Massage can help dissipate such stress, especially when used in conjunction with other stress reduction techniques such as deep breathing, progressive relaxation, proper nutrition, and lifestyle habits such as proper amounts of sleep and recreation. Some cases of emotional stress are best referred to psychotherapists.

Massage used in a stress reduction program will include techniques and qualities that evoke the relaxation response. The relaxation response is triggered by affecting the parasympathetic nervous system through the nerve endings in the skin and encouraging specific muscle relaxation and diaphragmatic breathing.

Apply massage to specific tight muscles and for general relaxation. The most effective techniques for general relaxation are long sliding movements and kneading. Techniques that tend to stimulate, such as percussions or frictions, should be avoided. Movement should be smooth and flowing, at a slow to medium pace, with light to moderate pressure.

The athlete should be encouraged to refrain from unnecessary talk during the session, focus on deep breathing, relax the body part being worked on, and to alternately focus on and then let go of tensions. A massage session is a good opportunity for the athlete to learn relaxation techniques.

The environment can play an important part in massage for general relaxation. Indirect light, quiet, and warmth enhance the relaxing effects of the massage. Whirlpool, sauna, steam, or taking a hot shower before the session may also enhance the effects of the massage.

REHABILITATION MASSAGE

Physical therapists, athletic trainers, massage therapists, chiropractors, and orthopedic physicians use massage as an effective addition to standard methods of sport injury rehabilitation. All injuries need some level of rehabilitation; for minor injuries exercise and massage may suffice. We define *rehabilitation massage* as massage applied specifically to severe injuries or conditions that disable the athlete and require the care of a physician, specifically injuries or conditions needing surgery or some form of systematic therapy designed to restore the injured part to its former capacity.

In rehabilitation, massage is one modality among many that form a complex system of recovery. Further, it is often the work of a health care team, rather than one individual, that brings about the greatest results in rehabilitation. The massage therapist assisting in rehabilitation works closely with the primary care physician and the athletic trainer or physical therapist.

It is clear that the promotion of early mobility as well as the reduction of pain, edema, and muscle spasm are major goals in rehabilitating sport injuries. We have witnessed the beneficial effects of individual massage techniques on exactly these conditions. However, there are no easy formulas for the use of massage with severe injuries.

We introduce this type of massage by offering a general philosophy and do not make any specific claims on how to perform rehabilitation massage. It is our intent to offer some stimulus for thought on using rehabilitation massage in presurgical and postsurgical situations and to discuss its effect on the formation of healthy scar tissue, return to normal ROM, relief of muscle tension, improved circulation, and reduced anxiety.

Massage Before Surgery

Many disabling conditions are treated conservatively prior to recommending surgery in the hopes that such treatment may avoid the need for surgery altogether. This conservative treatment may include any number of exercises, rest, hydrotherapy, various specialized electrical and rehabilitative equipment, and massage.

Massage may provide a better physiological environment for other modalities used in rehabilitation. For example, massage may be used to reduce muscle spasms in athletes suffering from disc disorders and allow easier use of traction devices that may resolve the condition without surgery. Massage may also be an adjunct to chiropractic treatment.

If surgery is needed after all, the athlete may have a more positive attitude toward surgery feeling satisfied that other avenues have been tried. Attitude is an important component of healing and recovery, and the relationship that develops between the therapist and the athlete during the presurgery massage sessions may help reduce the athlete's anxiety and prepare him or her mentally and emotionally for the procedure.

If the general health of the tissue prior to surgery has any effect on the recovery potential of that tissue after surgery, massage may be especially beneficial. Massage can improve circulation and reduce muscle spasm and splinting, thus providing a healthier, pliable, nutrient- and oxygen-rich tissue prior to surgery and perhaps improve the recovery potential of the tissues.

There is no evidence to support the notion that surgery should be withheld until massage is applied, but there may be enough evidence to consider including massage in any conservative treatment program or to consider prescribing it when surgery is scheduled weeks in advance.

Massage After Surgery: Acute Phase

In the acute postsurgical phase, massage will help reduce edema in the surrounding tissues, improve circulation and therefore cell nutrition, reduce muscle spasm, and provide an analgesic effect. Appropriate massage to the tissues surrounding the injury site and general relaxing massage to the entire body may relieve pain and irritation caused by the mechanical pressure of edema and the retention of metabolites due to immobility.

Massaging the injury site directly, or if infection is present or highly likely, is contraindicated in the acute phase. There is the risk of doing more harm than good following surgery, so massage must be applied with utmost caution and care. However, in the later phases, once the scar is healed and rehabilitation exercises have begun, more aggressive massage therapy may be applied.

Massage After the Acute Phase

After the acute phase has passed and the sutures are removed, massage will assist in recovery for the same reasons as in the acute phase. In addition, massage encourages movement, reduces soreness, helps develop healthy scar tissue, serves as reward motivation, and generally increases the athlete's sense of well-being.

As we discussed in chapter 1, massage aids the development of healthy, functional scar tissue, which is always a concern after surgery. Deep-transverse friction massage is the most common technique used for this purpose and may help reduce the risk of reinjury or the development of a chronic pain cycle at the site of the scar.

According to Arnheim and Prentice (1993) in their *Principles of Athletic Training*, "When an injured body is immobilized for a period of time, a number of disuse problems adversely affect muscle, joints, ligaments, bone, and the cardiovascular system." They also say, "Whenever possible, the athlete, without aggravating the injury, must continue to exercise the entire body" (p. 348).

The reduction of muscle soreness and spasm, as well as the direct anesthetic effect of massage, encourage movement. With less pain and greater ROM, the athlete is more likely to follow the prescribed rehabilitation exercises and may perform such exercises more effectively. Recovery sports massage is also used during rehabilitation to address the negative effects of rehabilitation "workouts." Patients may view massage as a reward for a good effort on the rehabilitation equipment, and the massage itself serves as valuable motivation. During intense rehabilitation exercises, athletes have been heard to say, "I'll do this only because I'm getting a massage tomorrow."

The psychological effects of massage are beneficial in the healing process. Massage may reduce anxiety over the outcome of the surgery and future athletic potential. In addition, the one-on-one attention, the time spent listening, and the caring touch expressed with massage often promote a greater sense of well-being, a better attitude, and perhaps a faster return to peak performance.

CHAPTER 4

SPORTS MASSAGE AT ATHLETIC EVENTS

Sports massage is given at competitive events (e.g., races, games, and tournaments) to help athletes prepare physically and mentally for performance, to reduce the potential for injury, and to facilitate recovery after or between performances. At events, massage is typically applied by athletes themselves, a coach, or a sports massage specialist.

How sports massage is utilized at events varies with the needs of the athletes, type of sport, team or individual preparation routine, and resources. For example, individual competition lends itself to all phases of event massage (pre-event, interevent, and postevent), but in team sports like football and basketball, the team's pregame and half-time routines usually preclude pre-event and interevent massage.

PRE-EVENT MASSAGE

Massage may be used within the 4 hours preceding an event to help the athlete achieve optimal physical and psychological readiness. Its application may be as simple as the athlete frictioning his or her own legs as part of a warm-up routine or may involve a short session with a sports massage specialist.

Massage may be used for purely physiological reasons (e.g., to oxygenate muscles by increasing circulation or to relax tight muscles and improve flexibility). Massage may also be used for its beneficial psychological effects: to reduce precompetition anxiety, to provide stimulation for "psyching up," or as part of an athlete's preparation ritual. As the body and mind of the whole athlete approach top functioning, performance potential increases.

To the extent that pre-event massage helps prepare the tissues for the stress that will be placed on them in the immediate competitive situation, it can be said to decrease injury potential. By aiding warm-up and relieving muscle tension, massage also helps prevent muscle pulls and tears.

Pre-Event Massage by Athletes

Athletes may use self-massage in a warm-up routine as an effective complement to stretching. Massage techniques such as compression, friction, and percussion are easily self-administered and help oxygenate tissues and raise tissue temperature. Direct pressure to stress points or acupressure points in areas to be stressed most in the upcoming activity can help make tissues more supple and enhance the effects of stretching (Meagher, 1990; Namikoshi, 1985). Light, rapid percussion stimulates nerves and improves alertness.

Self-Massage Warm-Up for Feet and Legs

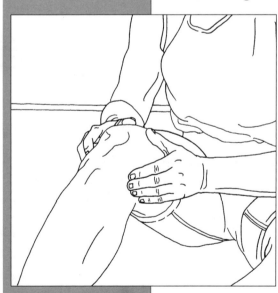

Figure 4.1
Self massage—
friction to the knee.

It is easy for athletes to incorporate self-massage techniques into their warm-up routines. These techniques are especially appropriate for athletes whose legs are stressed in their sports, such as runners, cyclists, and basketball players. As in all pre-event sports massage, the pressure is light to moderate and the pacing is brisk. Athletes can use the following self-massage techniques (see Figure 4.1 for an example).

- Direct pressure (thumb) on bottom of feet
- Direct pressure (fingertip, multiple digit) on top of feet
- Percussion (knuckles) on bottom of feet
- Compression of lower leg muscles (fingers)
- Friction (heel of hand) along tibialis anterior
- Friction (fingertip, multiple digit) around knee
- Compression (palmar) on quadriceps
- Jostling of quadriceps
- Percussion (beating) of quadriceps

Partner Warm-Up Massage for Upper Back, Shoulder, and Arm

There are simple yet effective massage techniques that athletes can apply to each other and that basically have the same purposes as self-massage. The advantages of partner massage are that some areas of the body can be reached more easily by another (e.g., upper back), the giver often has better leverage to exert more pressure, and athletes avoid stressing their own muscles in doing massage. Anxiety reduction is most effective if massage is given by another sympathetic person.

Massage by athletes can be done without oil, over clothes, in various positions (e.g., lying or sitting), and in many different locations (e.g., training room, hallways, locker room, or stands). Of course, oil may be used if desired, but it is not necessary, or appropriate in many cases, for pre-event massage (King, 1993).

Partner-massage techniques may be useful for athletes whose sports involve a lot of upper body activity, for instance, swimmers, power lifters, and tennis players. The pressure should be light to moderate and the pacing brisk. Partner-massage techniques include the following (see Figure 4.2 for an example).

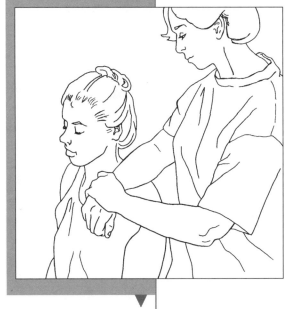

Figure 4.2
Partner massage—
compression on
the shoulders with
the forearms.

- Compression (forearm) on trapezius
- Kneading shoulders
- Direct pressure (elbow) along points on upper back
- Compression (multiple digit, squeezing) along the arm
- Jostling along length of arm
- Percussion (hacking) on upper back

Pre-Event Massage by Coaches

Coach-to-athlete pre-event massage uses the same techniques for warm-up as athlete-to-athlete pre-event massage. Team coaches are not likely to have much time to spend with an individual athlete and may use only a few simple techniques with some players.

A coach experienced in palpation may use some simple massage techniques to assess the condition of specific tissues that may need extra warm-up or a trip to the athletic trainer for some last minute treatment or wrapping. This scenario is most likely found in a one-to-one coaching situation in individual sports.

Massage may also be used by coaches in much the same way they use a slap on the back or hand on the shoulder to make physical contact and reassure an athlete before a performance. Massage provides an opportunity for acceptable nonthreatening touch, which may be applied while offering verbal encouragement and possibly last minute instruction.

Galen Describes Sports Massage in Ancient Rome

From 27 B.C.E. to 395 C.E. the Roman empire extended from Britain in the west to Asia Minor in the east and embraced much of the culture of ancient Greece. Massage was provided in the Roman baths (much like in the Greek *gymnasia*), and it was used to prepare athletes for competition and gladiators for ritual combat.

Galen (130-200 C.E.), a physician born in Asia Minor and steeped in ancient Greek culture, served as physician to prominent Romans. Early (157 C.E.) in his career he was appointed physician and surgeon to the gladiators; in this capacity, he supervised their diet and treated their wounds.

Galen's writings describe in some detail the methods used by the *aleitpes* (*anointers*, so called because they used oil) in their treatment of athletes, as well as the benefits of massage. In the following passage, Galen describes the *tripsis paraskeuastike* (i.e., massage before exercises):

> Hence, if anyone, immediately after undressing, proceeds to the more violent movements before he has softened the whole body, and thinned the excretions, and opened the pores, he incurs the danger of breaking or spraining some of the solid parts. There is danger also of the excretions, in the rush of moving spirits, blocking up the pores. But if beforehand you gradually warm and soften the solids and thin the fluids, and expand the pores, the person exercising will run no danger of breaking any part, nor of blocking up the pores. Hence, in order to secure this result, it is proper, by moderate rubbing with a linen cloth, to warm the whole body beforehand, and then to rub with oil. . . . And one should at first rub quietly, and afterwards gradually increasing it, push the strength of the friction so far as evidently to compress the flesh but not to bruise it. But it is not proper to apply such strong friction for a long time, but once or twice to each part; for we do not rub so as to harden the body of the boy, whom we are now training for the exercises, but to excite it to activity and augment its tone, and contract its porousness. . . . And in the imposition and circumflexion of the hands the rubbing should be very varied, and not merely directed from above to below, nor from below to above, but also slanting and oblique, transverse and sub-transverse . . . in order that all the fibres of the muscles, as completely as possible, may be rubbed. (Johnson, 1866, pp. 17-19)

Galen also describes *apotherapeia* (i.e., massage after exercises). In the following passage he recounts the benefits of this kind of massage to anyone who labors physically, to those who exercise for their health, and to athletes training for competition:

Its aim is double, viz, to empty the excretions, and to preserve the body from fatigue. . . . Now in the case of athletes, and indeed of those who dig, or take pedestrian exertion, or row, or go through any such toil necessary in daily life, weary pains (*kopoi*) occur more readily unless one has recourse to apotherapeia. . . . It is necessary indeed, to athletes, in order to prepare their bodies for the labours of the contest, which are sometimes immoderate and prolonged through the whole day, to undertake these consummating exercises. . . . But to those who exercise solely for the sake of health, it is neither necessary nor in any way useful to undergo excessive labours; so that there is no danger of their being seized with fatigue. But yet they ought to apply apotherapeia to their bodies, if not from expectation of fatigue, at least in order to empty the excretions. And it affords an additional security against fatigue. . . . For since the task is to effect an accurate evacuation of whatever residue of the excretions, warmed and rendered thin by the exercises, remain locked up in the solid parts of the body of the animal, it is proper to undergo rubbing by others. . . . Since, therefore, it is necessary at one and the same time to carry off the excretions and soften the tense parts, we must avoid the hard kinds of rubbing. . . . But since the rubbing must be [neither] slow nor hard, we must pour oil plentifully over the body of the person who is rubbed; for this contributes to both the quickness and softness of the rubbing; and it enjoys also another very great advantage, for it relaxes tension and softens the parts that have suffered in the more violent kinds of exertion. (Johnson, 1866, pp. 22-25)

The tradition of sports massage used by the Greeks and Romans was likely passed down informally by trainers to modern times. It is noteworthy that massage has maintained a long tradition in the very sports found in the ancient games, that is, track and field, boxing, and horse racing.

Pre-Event Massage by a Sports Massage Specialist

Specialists are called upon to achieve the greatest physical and mental benefits of sports massage. They also offer additional psychosocial support to the athlete and complement the work of coaches and athletic trainers, who typically do not have time to give pre-event massage.

Sports massage specialists may be called on to give pre-event massage to athletes they have been working with for months or years. A trainer or coach may alert the specialist to the unique preparation needs of certain athletes. For example, an athlete returning after rehabilitation may need special attention to warm-up a specific body part; another athlete may need more attention to flexibility of a certain joint to improve performance potential.

Sports massage specialists also provide pre-event massage at tournaments, races, and other events for athletes they have never massaged before. When the athlete is a stranger, sports massage specialists must plan the session on the spot, relying on information from the athlete and what their own hands tell them about the condition of the person.

A typical pre-event session includes a combination of various forms of compression, direct pressure, friction, and percussion applied to all major muscle groups as well as joint mobilization and stretching. This general massage is followed by specific work on the muscles and joints that will be used most in the upcoming event.

While there is some variation in expert opinion, there are some generally agreed upon guidelines for pre-event massage. According to these guidelines a pre-event massage session should

- be 15 to 20 minutes in duration,

- have an upbeat tempo,

- avoid causing pain,

- concentrate on the major muscle groups to be used in the upcoming performance,

- use techniques to increase circulation and joint movement (e.g., compression, direct pressure, friction, lifting and broadening, percussion, jostling, joint mobilizations, and stretching), and

- adjust for optimal psychological readiness (i.e., soothing for an anxious athlete and stimulating for most others).

Experienced sports massage specialists may make exceptions to the above guidelines. For example, athletes who receive massage frequently may want a deeper massage with attention to certain stress points that may cause pain. Other athletes may request that a session further away in time from the actual event be longer in duration; for example, a session 4 hours before an event may last 45 minutes instead of 15 minutes because it would not be part of the actual warm-up for the performance.

INTEREVENT MASSAGE

When an athlete is required to compete several times during a 1- or 2-day period, as in a track meet, or continuously over a several-day period, as in a cross-country bicycle race, interevent sports massage helps both recovery and preparation. It addresses the athlete's needs in the short periods between performances.

Interevent massage combines aspects of the pre-event and postevent applications. The athlete is recovering from one performance and preparing for the next one.

The session should generally be short and light (variation depending on the proximity of the next event) and focus on areas needing immediate attention. The specific goals of the session will depend on the unique needs of the athlete and the particular sport.

Improving circulation for metabolite removal and better cell nutrition is a priority. Less invasive techniques such as stretching and positional release are useful for tight areas. As in all event situations, avoid deep and painful techniques.

General guidelines for interevent massage suggest that the massage should

- be 10 to 15 minutes in duration,

- not include deep or painful work,

- focus on recovery of muscle groups used most,

- give attention to specific areas of tension from the preceding performance, and

- give attention to psychological recovery and readiness for the next performance.

Exceptions to the above recommendations might occur if the next event were several hours away, as in a swim meet, or the next day, as in a 5-day bicycle race. In the latter case, the massage session may last from 1 to 1-1/2 hours and include general relaxation techniques, for example, sliding strokes.

In the special case of a very short period of time between events, simple recovery techniques (e.g., kneading) applied without oil may be used on the most stressed muscles. A trainer kneading a boxer's shoulders between bouts is a familiar example.

As in the pre-event situation, interevent massage may be given athlete-to-athlete, coach-to-athlete, or by a sports massage specialist. Self-massage may be effective for the warm-up phase, but massage for recovery is best received from someone else.

POSTEVENT MASSAGE

Massage given within 4 hours after an event is used primarily to facilitate physical and psychological recovery. During postevent massage certain problem conditions may also be identified, evaluated, referred to other health care practitioners, or otherwise addressed.

Some general guidelines for postevent massage are that it should

- be of short duration (10-15 minutes) closer in time to the event and of longer duration (30-90 minutes) 1 hour or more after the event;

- feature lighter pressure, especially closer to the event time;

- give special attention to muscles stressed in the performance;
- utilize techniques known to facilitate metabolite removal, muscle relaxation, and general relaxation (e.g., compression, sliding strokes, kneading, jostling, positional release, joint mobilizations, and stretching); and
- include first aid or referral for problem conditions.

The athlete should cool down to a recovery heart rate, restore fluid balance, and do some light movement to facilitate metabolite removal before receiving postevent massage. Of course, an athletic trainer or other medical personnel should immediately evaluate suspected injuries.

Although self-massage can be beneficial in the postevent situation, the techniques used for recovery can be more easily applied by a partner, coach, or massage specialist. The athlete can also be more completely at rest during the massage. As in the pre-event massage, recovery techniques that do not use oil may be applied by another athlete or a coach.

Postevent Massage by a Sports Massage Specialist

The role of the sports massage specialist in the postevent situation includes both facilitating recovery and dealing with problem conditions. The extent to which problem conditions are dealt with depends on how close to the actual performance the massage session is and the availability of other health care professionals at the event.

A massage closer to the event time might include more first aid (e.g., muscle cramps), injury assessment, and referral. Although massage specialists are generally at low risk for coming into contact with blood-borne pathogens, exposure to blood occasionally occurs in postevent situations. Chafing, blood blisters, and road rash from falls are common at road races, triathlons, and bicycle events. Appendix A describes the application of universal precautions for sports massage at events. A massage therapist should also be alert to dehydration, hyperthermia, and hypothermia. When appropriate, athletes should be referred to an athletic trainer or medical team at the event.

The longer in time the massage session is from the event, the more likely medical emergencies will have been taken care of. In this case, recovery is the main focus. In the absence of medical problems, recovery massage is indicated, for example, light compression, sliding strokes, kneading, jostling, joint mobilizations, and stretching. Depth of pressure should be monitored carefully. Especially after long-distance events, muscles will be sore to the touch. Light pressure should be used, and deep-transverse friction should be avoided.

Hyperthermia and Hypothermia

Athletes may experience problems in maintaining a safe and comfortable core body temperature, particularly after long-distance events and in extreme weather. When greeting athletes for a postevent massage, you should assess the athlete's general condition, including visual observation and verbal interaction to detect signs of hyperthermia and hypothermia.

If you find the following conditions during postevent massage, the athlete should be treated with first aid or referred for medical attention.

Hyperthermia, having a body temperature much higher than normal, occurs when the body's rate of heat production exceeds its ability to dissipate the heat. Conditions that increase the potential for hyperthermia include high air temperature (above 99 degrees), high humidity, high altitude, and dehydration. Signs of hyperthermia include muscle cramps, clumsiness, stumbling, excessive—or no—sweating, headache, nausea, dizziness, apathy, and any gradual impairment of consciousness.

Loss of body fluids is a major factor in hyperthermia, and athletes should replace fluids adequately before receiving postevent massage. If athletes come for massage showing signs of hyperthermia, offer them more fluids. First aid should be given for the following conditions.

Muscle cramps (see directions for postevent muscle cramps on pages 72-73). If an athlete begins to have cramps in many different muscles throughout the body, pack the person in ice and get immediate medical attention.

Heat exhaustion. Symptoms of heat exhaustion include headache, nausea, hair erection on the chest and upper arms, chills, unsteadiness, fatigue, cool skin, and sweating. Do the following:

- Refer the athlete to medical personnel.
- While waiting for medical help, help administer first aid, including ice on the back of the neck and rest in cool shade. Have the athlete drink cool fluids and sit or lie near a fan.

Heat stroke. Symptoms of heat stroke include incoherent speech, confusion, aggressive behavior, unconsciousness, and the absence of sweating. Do the following:

- Refer the athlete to medical personnel immediately.
- Do not administer fluids by mouth.

Hypothermia, having a core body temperature much lower than normal, occurs when the body's rate of heat production is exceeded by its heat loss. Conditions that increase the potential for hypothermia include cool, wet, or rainy days and a high altitude.

Early signs of hypothermia include shivering, euphoria, the appearance of intoxication, and blue lips and nail beds. As the core temperature continues to fall, an athlete will become disoriented and may hallucinate, become combative, or lose consciousness. Do the following:

- Refer the athlete to medical personnel immediately; advanced hypothermia is an extreme medical emergency.
- While waiting for medical help, administer first aid by helping the athlete change into dry clothes, drink warm liquids, wrap the body in a blanket, cover the head, and move (e.g., walk or use passive joint mobilizations).

Relaxing Muscle Cramps

After the all-out effort of competition, especially in distance events, muscle cramping may occur. Dehydration can lead to muscle cramping, so before giving a sports massage, be sure that athletes have replaced fluids and electrolytes lost in physical exertion. If cramping occurs during postevent massage, offer the athletes more fluids. The following approaches, using the gastrocnemius muscle for illustration, may help return the cramping muscle to a relaxed state.

Direct Compression

Sustained pressure is applied to a muscle spasm with the full hand, a fist, forearm, or knee. Take the muscle in spasm off stretch before applying pressure.

Direct pressure

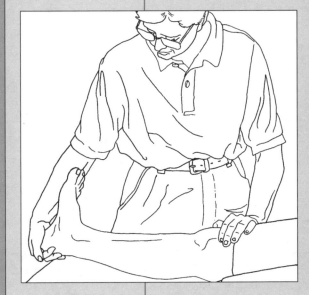

Mild Stretch

Use a mild static stretch of the cramping muscle.

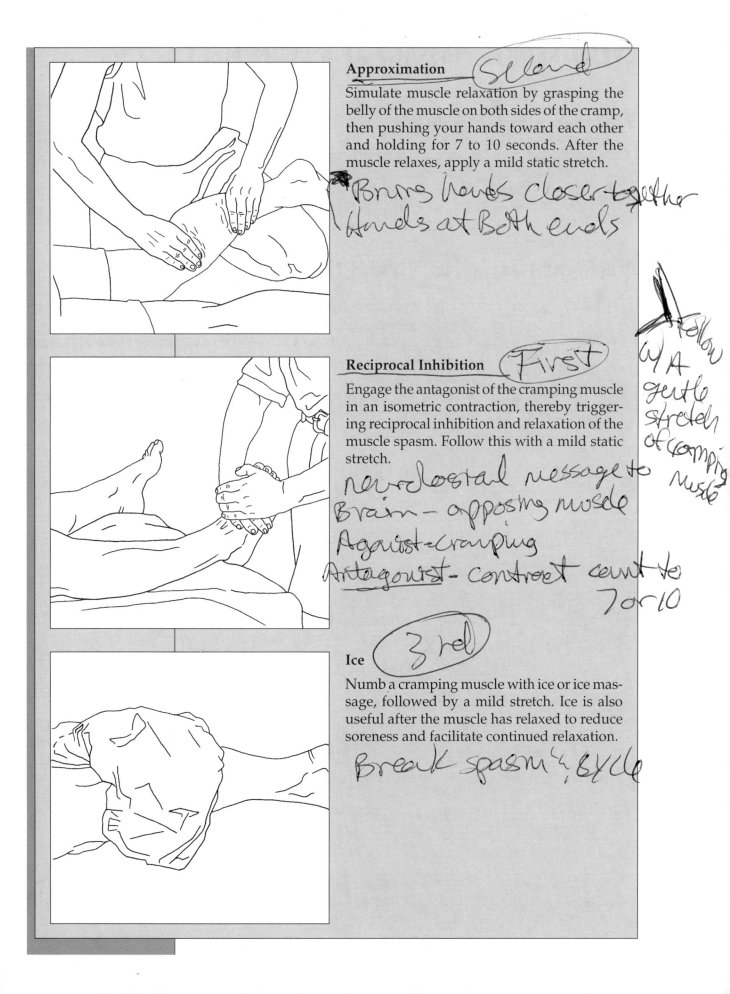

Approximation ~~Second~~

Simulate muscle relaxation by grasping the belly of the muscle on both sides of the cramp, then pushing your hands toward each other and holding for 7 to 10 seconds. After the muscle relaxes, apply a mild static stretch.

Bring hands closer together
Hands at Both ends

Reciprocal Inhibition ~~First~~

Engage the antagonist of the cramping muscle in an isometric contraction, thereby triggering reciprocal inhibition and relaxation of the muscle spasm. Follow this with a mild static stretch.

Follow w/ A gentle stretch of cramping muscle

neurological message to Brain - opposing muscle
Agonist - cramping
Antagonist - contract count to 7 or 10

Ice ~~3 rel~~

Numb a cramping muscle with ice or ice massage, followed by a mild stretch. Ice is also useful after the muscle has relaxed to reduce soreness and facilitate continued relaxation.

Break spasm & cycle

EVENT SPORTS MASSAGE AT A SWIM MEET

Sports massage is often provided at individual sporting events such as track and field and swim meets. Postevent massage may be arranged by the host school or event sponsor, and some teams travel with their own sports massage specialists.

The following sections describe how a university athletic department can provide sports massage for its swim team at away meets. They are based on a 1993 interview with Jill Bielawski, the massage therapist for the University of Arizona swim team.

Pre-Event Massage at a Swim Meet

The team typically arrives 2 days before an important meet to give the swimmers time to settle into their new surroundings. A massage room is set up at the team's hotel, and swimmers receive full-body massages that last from 30 minutes to 1 hour to help them calm down and begin to prepare for the meet. This massage employs moderately firm pressure and addresses trigger points, but no deep work (e.g., deep-transverse friction) is performed.

At the meet site, there is usually an area near the pool set aside for massage tables. On event day, the pre-event massage lasts from 10 to 20 minutes; its purpose is to help the swimmers get mentally prepared, focused, and psyched up and to enhance the warm-up by improving circulation. Images evoked include "getting things moving," feeling "as light as air," and "fluffing up" the muscles. Many believe that in the pre-event situation, the preparation for the swimmer is about 50% mental.

Pre-event massage for swimmers uses fast-paced sliding strokes, jostling, joint mobilizations, and stretching. Oil may be used because "many swimmers like the feel of the oil on their bodies—like gliding through water." No oil is applied to the feet or hands because of the safety hazard posed from slipping on the pool deck or blocks.

Sometimes swimmers wear a warm-up to prevent chilling while waiting for their events. In this case, massage is given over the warm-up and no oil is used. Compression techniques replace sliding strokes for stimulating circulation.

The areas of concentration in pre-event massage for swimmers vary depending on the swimmer's specific event. For example, in a pre-event massage for a freestyle swimmer the emphasis is on the arms and back with joint mobilizations and hip stretches. For the breast stroke, emphasis is on arms, neck, back, and legs, particularly the adductors and abductors.

Interevent Massage at a Swim Meet

Massage between swim-meet events is short (10-15 minutes) and fast paced. It is most often done over sweat suits to prevent chilling, and therefore oil is not commonly used. Care is taken to stimulate, not sedate, the swimmer. Compressions and sliding strokes, distal to proximal, enhance venous return.

Occasionally a muscle will have tightened up because of stress at the site of a previous injury. In that case, the massage may be deeper and more aggressive to relieve the restriction in movement and increase mobility. Ice may also be used in this case.

Postevent Massage at a Swim Meet

A postevent massage is often performed poolside over a sweat suit (to prevent chilling) and lasts about a half hour. At this point swimmers tend to be emotionally and physically exhausted.

Use light compressions, jostling, stretching, and joint mobilizations, and give special attention to areas stressed most during competition. Slow-paced movements facilitate general relaxation.

If the postevent massage is given in the makeshift hotel massage room, massage may be performed directly on the skin using oil, because the swimmers are less exhausted and the room can be kept warmer. Use sliding strokes for general relaxation and to improve venous return.

Between competitions, athletes continue to train and practice their skills. Chapter 5 describes how to use maintenance massage between competitions to help athletes maintain optimal physical and mental condition.

CHAPTER 5

MAINTENANCE MASSAGE

Maintenance sports massage refers to massage received by athletes on a regular basis as part of their training regimen. The purpose of maintenance massage is to help athletes maintain optimal physical condition during training.

Maintenance sessions include general recovery massage on the entire body with remedial massage in problem areas and extra attention to tight or sore muscles, stiff joints, and former injury sites. Afterward, athletes should feel relaxed, loose, and refreshed.

The emphasis will vary depending on the athlete and the particular sport. For example, the legs are most critical to a runner, cyclist, dancer, or skater, and the upper body will get more attention from a swimmer, tennis player, or gymnast.

Because the nature of a maintenance massage is so individual, there is no "typical" session. However, there are routines that can be used as a starting point. During a basic routine, when you come to a section of the body with a problem condition, simply spend more time on that area using techniques designed to treat the specific problem.

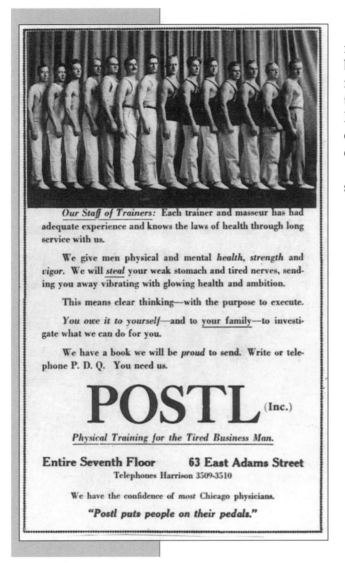

Chapter 3 offers a good example of a basic recovery routine that uses no oil or other lubricant. In this chapter, we outline a general recovery routine using oil that can serve as the basis for a maintenance sports massage. Methods for addressing specific problem conditions are found in chapter 3 in the section on remedial massage (pages 50-59).

General guidelines for maintenance massage are as follows. It should

- be scheduled regularly (i.e., once or twice a week or biweekly),
- last from 1/2 to 1-1/2 hours,
- include general recovery massage as a foundation,
- include remedial massage for problem conditions,
- give extra attention to the condition of areas commonly stressed in the athlete's sport,
- use a full range of techniques and methods of massage appropriate to session goals, and
- be moderate in tempo.

SAMPLE MAINTENANCE MASSAGE WITH OIL

The following section contains a sample routine for maintenance sports massage using oil. It is a basic recovery routine that can be modified to address the specific needs of each athlete.

Keep in mind that this is a general description only. It is impossible to describe every movement made during a massage session; no two sessions are exactly alike. The accomplished practitioner combines, blends, alternates, and otherwise varies movements to address specific conditions found in the tissues and joints during the session. The qualities of movement (pace, rhythm, pressure) will also vary with the situation. Use this routine as a model from which to practice general maintenance massage using oil.

The Gymnasia of Ancient Greece

Some of the earliest records of massage in the training of athletes are descriptions of the gymnasia in the ancient Greek cities of Athens and Sparta. Elite athletes of the ancient Olympic games, as well as the general citizenry who frequented the gymnasia, received massage as part of their training routines. Professional trainers (*paidotribes*) were often retired athletes who served in many capacities—including coach, masseur, nutritionist, physiotherapist, and hygienist. Sometimes specialists called *aleiptes*, or anointers (which alludes to the oil that was generously applied), did the massage during training and before and after competition. Many massage specialists were slaves.

In *The Anatriptic Art* (1866), Walter Johnson describes the routine at the ancient Greek gymnasium in which sports massage was an integral part:

> The youth was first rubbed by the paidotribes with oil; this process was called the preparatory rubbing—tripsis paraskeuastike. He then proceeded to some of the lighter exercises, as playing at ball; after which he sprinkled himself with Egyptian dust, and sought a companion (sungumnastes) to wrestle with. When sufficiently exercised, he passed into the room of the anointer (aleiptes), who by aid of the stlengis or strigil, as the Romans called it, helped him to scrape off his dust, oil, and sweat, and then rubbed him again with oil, which process was called apotherapeia. This done, he entered the warm bath, and after a short stay proceeded to the cold bath, and from the cold bath he returned to the alieptes who anointed him a second time, and sent him about his business. (p. 16)

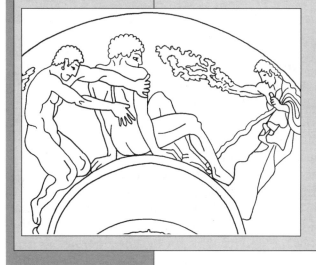

The gymnasium occupied a central place in Greek civic life, so that information from Greek medical science was available to trainers. Medical writers who frequented the gymnasium had personal contacts with trainers; medical writings about diet, exercise, muscle physiology, and hydrotherapy were reviewed and applied in training athletes.

Prone Position

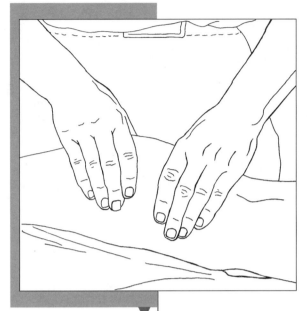

Figure 5.1
Kneading the muscles
of the lower leg.

Legs

The client is prone, and you are at the side of the table near the feet, facing the athlete's head. The session begins on the left leg with sliding movements. During the warming phase, apply sliding movements in long smooth strokes from the heels to the hip or waist. The hands are in palmar-overlay position and pressure begins very light and slowly deepens as the tissues become warmed. Apply more pressure on the movement toward the hip and less on the return to the ankle. The idea is to mechanically enhance venous return, but maintain contact on the return for continuity and relaxing effect.

After the warm-up, work the leg in parts from the hip to the ankle. Compression, deep sliding, broadening, and kneading are applied to the buttocks first, then the posterior thigh, then the lower leg. Knead the muscles of the lower leg as shown in Figure 5.1. End with a few more long sliding movements. Repeat the sequence for the right leg.

Back

Warm the back with compressions and long sliding movements from the shoulders to the waist. The hands are in full-palmar position to provide a broad contact surface. Be sure to massage laterally to include the sides and medially along either side of the spine. These movements may be repeated going from the waist to the shoulders.

Once the entire back is sufficiently warm and the skin begins to blush, begin more specific work. Starting with the upper shoulder area, apply compressions and then gentle kneading to the upper trapezius and levator scapula muscle in the area where the neck meets the shoulder. Apply some sliding movements to the back of the neck with your fingertips pulling from the shoulders to the occiput. Then work a bit more deeply with thumb slides to the rhomboids and trapezius between the scapula and the spine. Interrupt this with a few long sliding movements to the entire back, then return to the deeper work in the shoulder area. Once these tissues have softened a bit, apply gentle knuckling over the scapula to the infraspinatus muscle moving from the vertebral border toward the humerus.

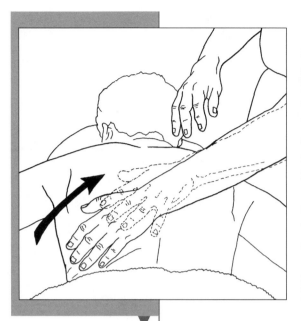

Figure 5.2
Full-palmar sliding
movement over the ribs.

Massage the rest of the thoracic region with thumb slides to the muscles that run along either side of the spine, first in the direction of the fibers in long movements up and down the side of the spine, then across the fibers in short movements from the spine out toward the side about an inch or two. Apply palmar slides over the ribs; push out from medial to lateral or pull in from the sides toward the spine as shown in Figure 5.2.

Massage the lumbar area in much the same way as the thoracic: Use thumb slides along the side of the spine and from the spine out all the way to the side.

A final application of palmar sliding movements from the shoulders to the waist completes the whole-back massage.

Supine Position

Legs

Before applying lubricant to the right leg, do some compressions to the thigh muscles. Rocking compressions not only relax the thigh but also mobilize and warm the hip joint and relax the entire leg, so these can be very helpful as a starting technique. Then apply oil and perform palmar sliding movements from the ankle to the hip.

When the thigh muscles are warmed up, the athlete is ready for some kneading movements and broadening (see Figure 5.3). These should be followed once again by deep-palmar slides from the knee to the hip.

The front of the lower leg is composed mostly of the large tibia (or shin bone) and is massaged along either side. Thumb slides work well here and can be followed by broadening done with the thumbs. Complete the shin with long palmar sliding movements from the ankle to the knee, pressing along either side of the bone.

Massage the ankle with fast-moving superficial friction or fingertip sliding movements all around the ankle bones. Apply sliding movements to both the dorsal and plantar surfaces of the foot, moving from the toes to the ankle. Figure 5.4 illustrates how to use the fingertips to massage between the bones of the dorsal foot.

Mobilize all the joints from the hip to the toes to conclude the work on the leg, then repeat the same sequence on the left leg.

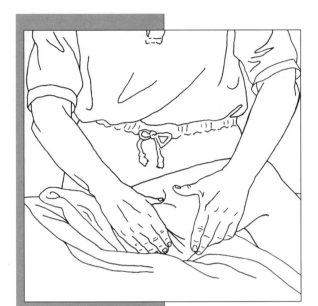

Figure 5.3
Kneading the adduc-
tors on the medial
side of the thigh.

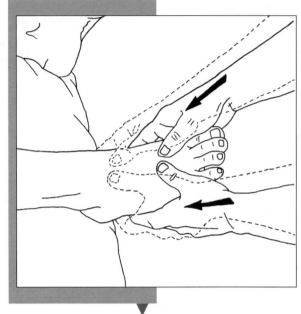

Figure 5.4
Fingertip sliding
movement on the
dorsal side of the foot.

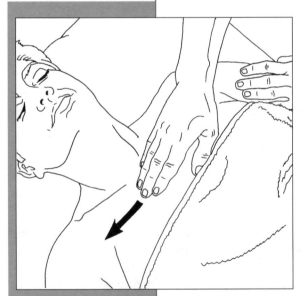

Figure 5.5
Full-palmar sliding
movement on the
pectorals.

Chest

Massage the chest with sliding movements on the pectoral muscles. Use your palm or the fingertips; begin with light pressure and gradually work deeper (Figure 5.5). Do not massage into the breast tissue; this massage should be applied to the upper portion of the chest only.

Arm and Shoulder

Begin with the arm pronated, palm down, on the table. You are at the side facing the athlete's head. Apply compressions along the entire arm. While using one hand to stabilize the arm at the wrist, apply one-handed palmar sliding movements, moving from the wrist to the shoulder. Lift the arm up by the hand and have the athlete completely relax it, then "wag" the arm by gently shaking it back and forth; this action will mobilize the shoulder.

Massage the upper arm with kneading and sliding movements from the elbow to the shoulder. Use your thumbs to perform broadening movements and deep thumb slides. Remember, all movements should be in the direction of venous flow (toward the shoulder).

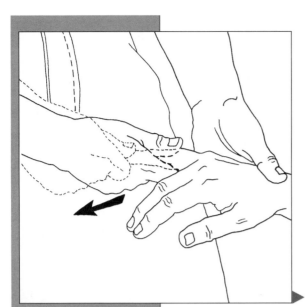

In addition apply deep thumb slides to the forearm from the wrist to the elbow, being sure to work on all sides of the arm.

Hand massage is similar to foot massage, with sliding movements on both the dorsal and palmar surfaces. Massage the athlete's fingers between your thumb and forefinger, pulling the finger slightly as you slide down as shown in Figure 5.6.

Finally, mobilize each joint by moving it through the ROM.

Figure 5.6   Sliding movement along the fingers.

Neck

Stand behind the athlete's head. Sliding movements are pulled from the shoulder to the head on either side, or both sides simultaneously. Move the neck through a passive ROM by lifting the head and gently moving it from side to side and stretching it into flexion. End the session with a slight traction of the neck. Hold the head in your palms, fingers grasping lightly under the occipital ridge, and pull gently back as shown in Figure 5.7. Release the traction after about 15 seconds, and continue to hold the head for about 10 more seconds. Slowly pull your hands away to end the session.

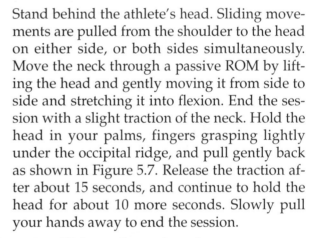

Figure 5.7   Slight traction to the neck.

COMMON MAINTENANCE PROBLEM AREAS

As you move from section to section during a general maintenance massage, you will encounter problem spots that need more detailed attention. These are usually tight, stiff, or sore areas. These problems commonly result from repetitive use, past injuries, or improper sports techniques.

These problem spots require additional recovery work (i.e., more time on the area) and some specific remedial massage. Techniques commonly used to address maintenance problem areas include deep friction, trigger-point work, direct pressure, and stretching.

Legs and Hips

Athletes most prone to leg and hip problems include runners, skiers, cyclists, karate and other martial artists, and soccer players. Deep friction and direct pressure on tendons, trigger-point work, and stretching at the ankle, knee, and hip are often helpful.

Back

Because both upper and lower body movements involve the back, athletes in most sports experience tension and soreness in this area. Compression, circular friction, and direct pressure are easily applied to the large muscles of the back.

Arms, Chest, and Shoulders

Athletes prone to upper body problems include gymnasts; tennis and other racquet sport players; judo and other martial artists; golfers; and volleyball, baseball, and softball players. Certain field events like discus, shotput, and javelin also stress the upper body.

Deep friction and direct pressure on tendons, trigger-point work, and stretching at the shoulder are often helpful. Compression and kneading can induce greater circulation.

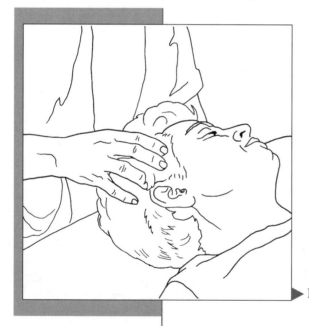

Neck and Head

The neck and head are sometimes forgotten as areas of tension except in sports like wrestling and American football. Massage can also relieve tension headaches caused by anxiety and stress. Circular friction and direct pressure on the neck and along the base of the skull, and on the head itself, especially on the frontalis and temporalis, help relieve tension in these areas (see Figure 5.8).

Figure 5.8   Friction to the temporalis.

Maintenance massage is the most comprehensive form of sports massage because it involves both general recovery and remedial work. Chapter 6 explains in more detail how to plan and give sports massage, including maintenance massage.

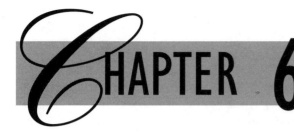

CHAPTER 6

PLANNING AND GIVING SPORTS MASSAGE

All massage sessions are individualized and require some advance planning. An experienced massage specialist can sketch a general plan quickly, but a beginner or student needs to think things out more carefully.

Many of the specific details of giving a massage emerge during a session as the giver interacts with the receiver. Qualities such as pressure, rhythm, pacing, and specificity are determined on the spot as the massage progresses. The details are altered as the receiver reacts to the massage and a clearer picture of what is called for develops in the session.

When you give a massage, you must also be able to handle the physical objects that are part of massage, such as bolsters, sheets, and towels. In addition, you need to employ good body mechanics to give a massage with ease.

PLANNING A SESSION

Just as the coach develops a game plan before a competition, you should plan individual sports massage sessions just prior to the session. Planning

Advice From Mat Bullock

Mat Bullock, athletic trainer for the University of Illinois, devoted an entire chapter of his book *Athletic Training Methods* (1925) to massage. Wanting to bring together "the knowledge and methods of the modern athletic trainer" (preface), Bullock utilized his 11 years of experience as trainer at the university (1914–1925).

Bullock used the classic French terminology to describe massage techniques: *effleurage*, *friction*, *petrissage*, and *tapotement*. He avoided giving set massage routines; he realized that a trained masseur would vary his approach, depending on the desired results.

He advised students to watch or help a trained masseur, but he encouraged them also to develop their own techniques while following fundamental rules. He wrote:

> A good masseur thinks less of the manner of moving his hands than of the tissues upon which he is working. Therefore, the trainer who would have his massage be effective must have a good general knowledge of anatomical structure and a thorough understanding of the special conditions in the individual upon whom he is working. (p. 16)

Bullock further commented on how to plan a massage session by choosing techniques to get the desired effects and tailoring the session to match the condition of the athlete on the table. He advised:

> In general the trainer can have no definite rule as to the duration and order of the movements, but should govern his massage by the condition of the athlete and the effects he desires to create, having in mind all the while that effleurage [sliding movements] chiefly causes relaxation; friction generates heat; and that tapotement [percussion] mainly promotes tone, and is occasionally used to end the massage. (pp. 20–21)

Bullock's manual (1925) lists a broad range of benefits of using massage in athletics, which include aiding in the recuperation of fatigued athletes; serving as a sedative or quieting influence on very nervous athletes; having a stimulating effect on tired athletes, those with phlegmatic temperaments, or those on the verge of becoming stale; relaxing athletes who need to rest (in the interval between events or between halves of a grueling game); and as a therapeutic agent. He regarded massage as beneficial in general training, before and after events, between events, and in treating injuries.

Bullock acknowledged that "massage is one of the most valuable phases of knowledge to the athletic trainer," but he warned against valuing it too highly. He urged that it be used "only when beneficial results are assured," and cautioned that "if overdone, [it] might tend to 'baby' the athletes and cause . . . a dependence on massage all out of proportion to its benefits" (p. 15).

involves determining the goals of the session, choosing appropriate techniques, and sequencing. These plans are usually executed within the context of a general pattern or massage routine. Table 6.1 lists the elements of a session plan and general considerations for each element.

Table 6.1	Elements of Planning a Sports Massage Session	
	Elements	**Considerations**
	Session goals	General goals Individual goals
	Choosing techniques	Primary effects desired Secondary effects desired
	Sequence of techniques	Beginning and end of session Effects of combination and order Preparing area for specific work
	Routine	Appropriateness for application Variation for individuals
	Environment	Adequate space Equipment and supplies Comfort of the athlete

Session Goals

Sports massage is "results oriented" and always has specific goals that are directly related to the athlete's performance and well-being.

The goals of any one session are determined by the timing of the session in relation to the athletes' training or competition schedule; their physical and emotional condition; and their immediate needs as determined by either the athletes themselves or the coach, athletic trainer, other health care professional, or massage specialist. Each session has a general purpose depending on where it falls in the training–competition cycle and is tailored to the individual athlete's situation.

Figure 6.1 shows a simple trouble-spots body chart that can be used to identify and record problem areas of individual athletes. Before a session begins, ask the athlete to mark areas of tightness, pain, or past injury on the chart to provide a quick reference and planning tool for the session.

Because of its individualized aspect, a session's goals may change at any time during the session. The better the massage specialist knows the athlete, the easier it is to plan an appropriate and effective session. The following list contains important questions that must be answered in planning a sports massage session:

- Is this a maintenance, pre-event, interevent, or postevent situation?

- What is the optimal physical condition for performance in this sport or event?

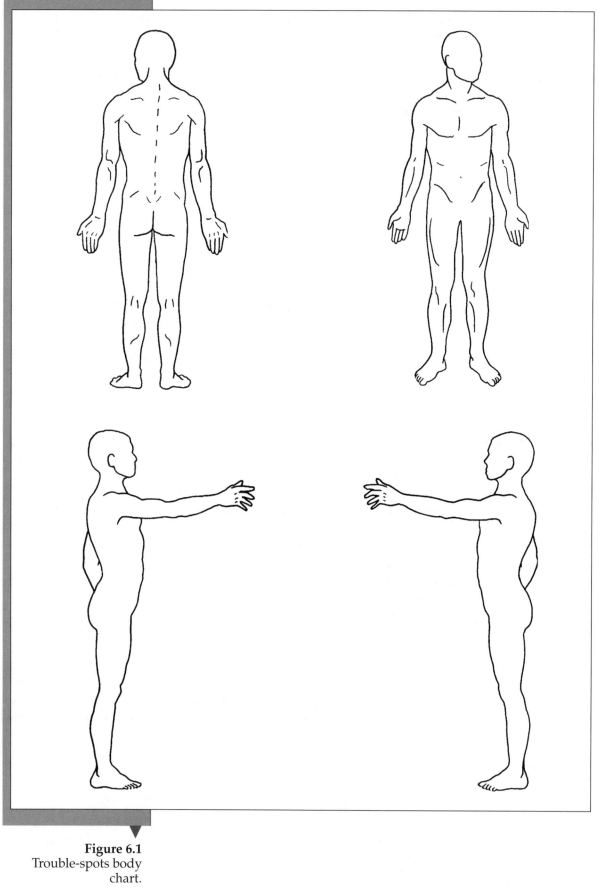

Figure 6.1
Trouble-spots body
chart.

- Which part of the athlete's body will be (have been) stressed most in this sport or event?

- Is there a specific problem condition or past injury site that needs to be addressed?

- What is the athlete's emotional state? What is appropriate for this time in relation to training or competition? Should the athlete be more stimulated or relaxed?

- What are the athlete's requests or complaints?

- What are the coach's, athletic trainer's, and health care professional's requests or directions?

With the above questions in mind, the specific goals of the session may be determined and prioritized. The plan tries to achieve the determined goals within the time available.

Choosing Techniques

The prioritized goals of the massage session determine which massage and related techniques are used, for how long, and in what order. Be aware of the primary and secondary effects of various techniques and combinations of techniques and choose the ones that will best achieve your goals.

For example, deep stroking, kneading, and compression facilitate general recovery. A combination of deep stroking and stretching increases flexibility. Deep-transverse friction breaks adhesions. Deep sliding strokes enhance circulation. Compression promotes durable hyperemia.

The more experience you have with a wide variety of techniques, the more effective you can be in planning and executing a successful sports massage session. You will be continually creating variations of techniques as you work, and you may acquire new methods with further instruction.

Sequence of Techniques

The sequence of techniques can have a great effect on the outcome. A session usually begins with general techniques such as sliding strokes over a large area, then moves on to working on specific areas or problems such as frictioning tendons around the knees and ankles, and then back to general work like percussion over the back and back of the legs to finish a session.

Sequencing may also involve using one technique to prepare for or to follow up another. For example, general compression and kneading may be used to prepare an area for more specific work on a particular muscle or muscle group, followed by stretches to help reeducate a muscle to its increased length.

Connecting strokes are used after work on a specific area to enhance the awareness of the body as a whole. Some movements help create a smooth transition from one body section or subsection to another (see Table 6.2).

Table 6.2	General Routine Sequence and Use of Specific Massage Techniques
General warm-up	Long sliding movements
	Compressions
	Kneading
	Superficial skin friction
	Joint mobilizations
Specific work	Deep friction
	Vibration
	Digital compression
	Thumb slides
	Positional release
	Stretching
	Skin rolling
Connecting	Long sliding movements
	Percussion
Transition	Long sliding movements
	Joint mobilizations

The Routine

There are no set formulas for sports massage—only general guidelines. Individuals giving massage typically establish a routine or general pattern of working that they customize for each athlete they work on.

You may have a different routine for maintenance and pre-event, interevent, and postevent sessions. You may also favor techniques that are uniquely suited to your physical capabilities or personality and that are especially effective for you. Your routine will change as you become more experienced and learn new techniques.

The elements of a sports massage routine are

- the sequence of positions,
- the sequence of sections and subsections worked on for each position, and
- the sequence of steps within each section.

The athlete's position may be supine, prone, side-lying, or sitting. A routine may include one or more positions in any order.

For each body position, determine the sequence of general sections to be addressed, that is, the arms, legs, back, neck, front torso, and head. Any sequence may be used; however, there are some common patterns. For example, in the prone position, you might work on the legs first, then the back. In the supine position, the sequence might be legs, arms, front torso, neck, and head. The sequence for the side-lying position might be legs, arms, and back. The upper body is usually addressed in the sitting position working back first, then arms, neck, and head (see Table 6.3).

Massage subsections within each general section of the body in a specific order. For example, prepare the whole arm with sliding movements or compressions, and then address smaller areas in order, from

Table 6.3	**Sample Positions and Sequence of Body Sections Used in Planning a Sports Massage Routine**	

Position	Sequence of Body Sections
Prone	Legs, back
Supine	Legs, arms, front torso, neck, head
Side-lying	Legs, arms, back
Sitting	Back, arms, neck, head

Table 6.4	**Section and Subsection Sequences Commonly Used in a Sports Massage Routine**	

Section	Subsection Sequence
Arm	Shoulder, upper arm, elbow, forearm, hand
Leg	Hip, thigh, knee, lower leg, foot
Back	Sacroiliac, lumbar, thoracic, shoulder girdle, neck
Head	Face, jaw, cranium, neck

the shoulder to the upper arm, elbow, lower arm, wrist, and hand. Working in subsections increases the specificity of the massage. Table 6.4 lists sample sequence patterns for general body sections.

Routines may vary from person to person, but once you have established a working routine, you will usually stay with it for a time. These routines create a foundation for the variations that address the specific needs of an athlete on any particular day.

Environment

The plan for a sports massage session should consider the environment whenever possible. The session frequently occurs in a locker room, training room, or at an event site, and ideal conditions are often out of the massage specialist's control. Besides having equipment and supplies, it is important to have enough space and, depending on the goals, relative quiet. Even the color of the room, feel of the table (whether it is soft or hard, or stable or loose), and availability of music can affect the outcome of the session.

GIVING SPORTS MASSAGE

Besides planning the session and setting up the environment, other aspects of the implementation of the massage deserve attention. These include choosing the right lubricant, the quality of the movements, general mechanics, body mechanics, and monitoring progress through feedback and pain.

Use of Oils and Other Topical Substances

Oils and other substances are commonly applied topically during sports massage for a number of reasons. One reason is simply to allow the hands to slide across the skin without irritating it. Various oils are good for this purpose, and individual practitioners have personal preferences usually based on the "feel" of the oil, for example, its lightness or thickness. Both vegetable and mineral oils are used.

Baumgartner and Athletic Massage After WW II

Albert Baumgartner, a former trainer at State University of Iowa, wrote *Massage in Athletics* in 1947. One of the first books written entirely about sports massage, it describes the techniques of classic Western massage, combining Swedish massage with the the techniques developed by the German J.B. Zabludowski (1851–1906).

According to Baumgartner, athletic massage is used for three general purposes:

> It is used as a *preparatory* or a preliminary massage to stimulate the body before a work-out or before competition. It is applied as an *intermediate* massage to maintain body energy and freshness during rest periods in practice or competition. The effect of massage in this case is that of a sedative. A third application is the *reconditioning* or recuperation massage performed after a work-out to revitalize the body. (pp. 8-9)

Baumgartner suggested that massage can have many different psychological effects, depending on the techniques applied and the content and quality of communication between the masseur and the athlete.

> It is important that we bear in mind the temperament of the individual athlete. In the preparatory massage, for instance, the hot-headed or ardent athlete with a strong starting fever should be given only a light muscle massage of the extremities, while the phlegmatic athlete should be massaged more vigorously. . . . A good massage is half of the athlete's preparation. (p. 5)
>
> The masseur, besides having technical ability, must be a good mind-reader, in order to understand the temperamental characteristics of his subjects. . . . During the massage it is easy to instill and divert courage. Upon this foregoing attribute rests the main reason for the popularity of many masseurs. (p. 101)

Baumgartner believed that "any sports trainer should be a well qualified masseur" and that "the athletic masseur should come from the ranks of professional masseurs or from the ranks of the sports teachers." He alluded to a lack of esteem for athletic masseurs and admonished that "a physical education instructor should not think himself too refined to enter the profession of the athletic masseur" (p. 11).

The athletic masseur as Baumgartner knew him had essentially disappeared by the early 1960s. The art was lost from physical education until it was revived in the 1970s within the ranks of professional massage therapists.

Common vegetable oils used for massage are olive, coconut, peanut, safflower, grape seed, and almond. Oils are often mixed to achieve the desired texture and performance, and several premixed oils for sports massage are available.

Sometimes small amounts of essential oils extracted from various plants, and thought to have special qualities, may be mixed with a base oil. The science of using essential oils is well developed in Europe and is called *aromatherapy*. In France aromatherapy is a medical specialization practiced only by licensed physicians (Tisserand, 1977).

Essential oils may be used for such effects as enhancing relaxation, stimulation, or healing. Arnica is one oil popular for its healing qualities.

Astringents such as witch hazel and rubbing alcohol are sometimes used to stimulate the skin and close pores. They may also be used to remove oil after massage.

Rubefacients are popular for the warm sensation they produce on the skin due to increased local circulation. Their benefit for deep penetrating heat is questionable, and they may irritate some athletes. Popular rubefacients on the market for athletes include Ben-Gay and Tiger Balm. Active ingredients often include camphor and eucalyptus. Herbal rubefacients include black pepper, juniper, and rosemary.

Various ointments and salves that are valued specifically for their healing qualities in treating sprains, bruises, and inflammations may be applied during sports massage. In addition to common medical ointments, there are some effective homeopathic ointments, such as Traumeel. Sometimes powders such as corn starch are preferred to prevent skin abrasion.

You can enhance the effects of the session by carefully choosing the substances you use. As always, what is used may vary with the needs of the situation and the preferences of the athlete and the therapist.

It should be noted that sports massage is often given without oil or any other topical substance, particularly in pre-event and interevent situations. Some techniques, such as deep friction and compression, usually work better without lubrication.

Qualities of Movement

The most important qualities of movement to consider when giving massage include pressure, rhythm, pacing, continuity, specificity, and sequence. Variations in these qualities help determine the physiological and psychological effects and effectiveness of the technique. Table 6.5 lists the qualities of movement important when giving massage and the general parameters of their variations.

Pressure

The pressure used with any technique should be appropriate for the body part or type and condition of tissue receiving massage. Pressure may vary from light on sensitive areas to moderate on normal tissues to heavy when working on problems such as chronic tightness. Working on a sore area with heavy pressure might cause tissue damage or "bracing" and should be avoided, and working too light may have little effect (see "Optimal Therapy Zone" on page 97).

Table 6.5	Variations in the Quality of Movements in Massage	
	Quality	Variations
	Pressure	Light to heavy
	Rhythm	Even or uneven
	Pacing	Slow to fast
	Continuity	Smooth or choppy transitions
	Specificity	General area to specific structure
		General to individual application

During a session, a part should first be warmed up or prepared with lighter pressure; gradually increase the pressure as you work. This allows the person receiving massage to adapt to the touch of the therapist and prepares the tissues for more vigorous movement—much like a warm-up in athletics.

Rhythm, Pacing, and Continuity

The rhythm and pacing of the movements are important to establish continuity and flow and have great effect on whether the technique is relaxing or stimulating to the athlete. For example, fast-paced percussion or swift, alternate sliding movements can be stimulating; slower kneading or smooth sliding movements are more relaxing.

Smooth transitions from one technique to another aid continuity. Once contact is made with the body, it should be broken very carefully to avoid "startling" the athlete or causing an uncomfortable feeling that may disrupt the effects of the massage.

Specificity

Specificity refers to the size of the area being massaged and whether the effects are general or local to a specific structure or small area. The smaller the area and more local the effects, the more you are said to be working with specificity.

Some techniques such as compression generally increase circulation to a wide area (less specificity), while cross-fiber friction or direct pressure on a trigger point might address a 1/2-inch square spot (more specificity). Figure 6.2 shows specific work on the ankle.

The ability to work with specificity comes with experience and knowledge; it is the product of knowledge of anatomy, the ability to palpate small or subtle conditions, and skill in certain massage techniques.

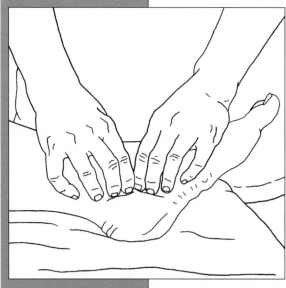

Figure 6.2
Specific work on the ankle.

General Mechanics

General mechanics refers to things like proper draping, use of towels and sheets, the use of pillows and other bolstering devices, and skill in changing client position. Proper draping allows the therapist to work unencumbered while preserving the modesty of the athlete. Besides being considered unethical, exposure of an athlete's genitals, gluteal cleavage, and breasts can cause uneasiness and prevent the athlete from relaxing or focusing. In sports massage the therapist frequently works through clothing or on top of a drape, which also requires some skill.

Towels and sheets are used to drape or when applying cold or heat and may be used rolled up as bolsters for positioning. Pillows and other devices are also used to help position clients to relieve stress on certain areas. Figure 6.3 shows typical draping for a female athlete, and Figure 6.4 illustrates the use of bolsters for support.

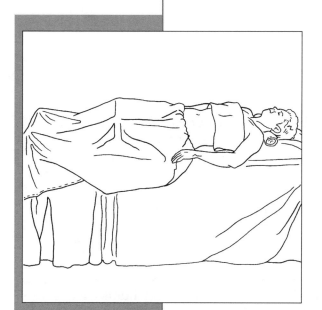

Figure 6.3
Draping for a
female athlete.

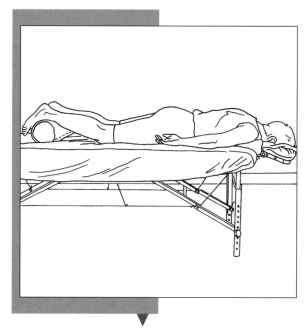

Figure 6.4
Use of bolsters for
support in the prone
position.

Although the common image of receiving a massage is one of lying prone or supine on a table, there are many positional variations including lying on the side and sitting (see Figures 6.5 and 6.6). It is useful for the massage therapist to be able to work with the athlete in a variety of positions. When athletes must change position, for example, from prone to supine, supine to side-lying, or prone to sitting, they can be guided to minimize awkwardness and possible "undoing" of the effects of the massage treatment.

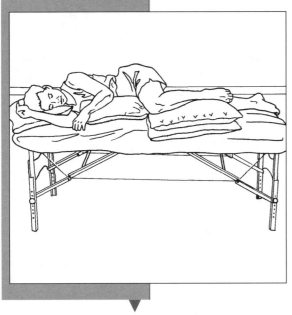

Figure 6.5
Side-lying position.

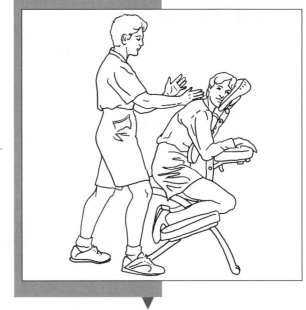

Figure 6.6
Sitting position using
a chair designed for
massage.

Body Biomechanics

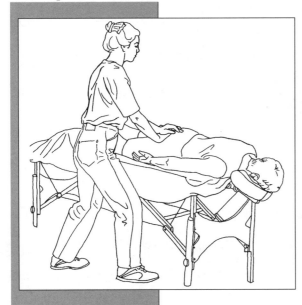

Figure 6.7
Good posture for
giving massage.

The body mechanics of the massage giver deserve special attention. Just as the athlete can develop physical problems because of poor posture and biomechanics, you can damage your own body by the way you use it while giving massage. The most common problems are thumb and wrist problems, various sites of tendinitis, and chronic tension in the back and neck. Figure 6.7 shows good posture for giving massage.

In general, it is best to keep the back straight, knees bent, wrists straight, and thumbs in line with the wrists while applying deep pressure. During pumping compression, it is helpful to use the hand-over-hand position to keep pressure off the wrists. An alternative hand position for compression is to use the back of a loose fist, which keeps the wrist straight and avoids strain.

Monitoring Progress and Pain

While giving massage, you get feedback on how the athlete is responding to the session in a number of ways. You can receive feedback through palpation, the feel of movement as in "end feel" of stretching, the athlete's answers to questions, and also the athlete's reaction to pain on movement or pressure.

Monitoring pain is one of the most valuable avenues of feedback. Pain is especially important because it may be an indication of damage to the tissues, and therefore, contraindication to certain kinds of techniques or qualities of movement. Athletes can learn to distinguish "good pain" and "bad pain" much as they do while working out or performing.

Different people have different emotional responses to pain. Some brace or tighten muscles against pain, which can be counterproductive in massage. Some are stoic and give no apparent feedback; they will sustain damage to tissues before saying anything.

Some theories say avoid pain altogether. This is especially true for event massage and general recovery. For remedial and rehabilitation situations, some experts believe that pain indicates that a therapeutic benefit is taking place. The optimal therapy zone theory describes how to monitor pain in the latter situation.

Optimal Therapy Zone

The concept of the *optimal therapy zone* (OTZ), developed by Scott Lamp (1989), is very useful in certain remedial and rehabilitation situations. The OTZ can best be described as an amount of pressure. Actually, it is the depth at which the therapist must work to be effective in certain situations; that depth is most easily described by the amount of pressure needed to reach it.

The OTZ is typically found when the pressure is enough to cause some discomfort, but not enough to cause voluntary or involuntary splinting of the area being worked on. The therapist must remain sensitive to the amount of pain the athlete is experiencing to avoid using too much pressure in an effort to get quick results. It is like trying to erase a mistake on a piece of paper—not enough pressure and it will not erase, too much and the paper tears.

Working in the OTZ has been found to be effective when the goal of the treatment is one of the following:

- Removal of chronic muscle hypertonicity
- Formation of healthy scar tissue
- Healing of tendinitis
- Breaking up of adhesions
- Deactivation of trigger points
- Increase in flexibility and range of motion
- Healing of subclinical muscle–tendon problems
- Prevention of problems resulting from biomechanical stress associated with an injury or muscle imbalance

Each athlete has his or her own OTZ, and each part of the body may have a different OTZ. The OTZ is not a set amount of pressure, but is determined by several factors related to the location, nature of the injury, and nature of the athlete.

Some areas of the body have more nerve endings than others and may therefore be more sensitive to touch or pressure. The presence of adipose tissue seems to decrease the pain tolerance level and increase the chance of delayed soreness after treatment. Adipose tissue also bruises more easily.

An athlete in good condition will typically have a higher pain tolerance than the norm for the general population. The more extensive the injury, however, the lower the pain tolerance. If the athlete is sick with a cold or flu, depressed, or worried, the pain tolerance decreases.

The level of confidence in the therapist also seems to have an effect. When athletes are unsure of the therapist's skill or unsure that the therapist is concerned about their pain experience, the level of apprehension rises while pain tolerance tends to drop.

Finally, the athletes' need or desire to recover quickly may result in higher pain tolerance. If their ability to perform affects their livelihood, self-esteem, or peer acceptance, the desire to recover can outweigh an otherwise lower pain tolerance. The concept of OTZ includes using appropriate massage techniques. Using inappropriate techniques for the situation or applying techniques improperly may result in pain with little or no benefit. Inappropriate techniques may also cause additional injury to the area.

Massage techniques most commonly used while working in the OTZ include deep-transverse friction, deep-digital pressure, deep thumb slides, and compression broadening movements. These may be applied while the athlete is completely relaxed or during active movement of the part being treated.

Treatment within the OTZ should never be longer than 10 minutes, and may be as short as 30 seconds. The therapist should move in and out of the OTZ and alternate techniques to give some relief from the discomfort. If the athlete's pain tolerance begins to decrease significantly, treatment in the OTZ should be discontinued for that session.

Sports massage therapists working in the OTZ should be knowledgeable about working with injuries, ice modalities, and deep-massage techniques. They should have good communication skills to explain the treatment and listen for signs of apprehension. They should be empathetic and supportive.

A "ruthless compassion" is needed to encourage the athlete to accept the treatment in the face of pain. Aggressiveness, but not overzealousness, is appropriate. The therapist must be in control, but allow the athlete to have the final word about when enough is enough.

Finally, the therapist must exhibit confidence. Remember, apprehension on the part of athletes seems to lower their pain tolerance and therefore the effectiveness of the work.

Athletes may experience soreness the day after the treatment. However, they should not feel severe soreness or exhibit any bruising, which would indicate that too much pressure was used. The therapist can minimize this delayed soreness by applying some general massage techniques or ice therapy to the area to soothe the nerves.

The athlete's report on the day following treatment can help the therapist determine the degree of success in working within the OTZ. We recommend that the therapist communicate with the athlete the day after the treatment.

Why work in the OTZ if it typically causes discomfort? The answer is that it gives faster results, a quicker return to optimal function, and less time away from training.

Chapters 1 through 6 have presented the basics of why, when, and how to give an effective sports massage. In chapter 7, we tackle the nuts-and-bolts issues of how to make it all happen by implementing a sports massage program in a variety of settings.

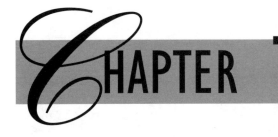

CHAPTER 7

IMPLEMENTING A SPORTS MASSAGE PROGRAM

Once you are convinced of the value of massage for enhancing the athlete's well-being and performance, you must decide how to implement a sports massage program. How do you find the resources? Do you hire a sports massage specialist? How do sports massage specialists interact with coaches, athletic trainers, and team physicians? Where do you find the time and space? Who gets massage? How often? For what purpose?

School and university athletic departments, elite amateur and professional athletic organizations, and organized athletic event sponsors, health clubs, and private clinics all provide sports massage services. Each setting has a unique set of circumstances to consider when implementing its program. This chapter considers the unique requirements for a variety of settings.

SCHOOL AND UNIVERSITY PROGRAMS

Some school or university athletic programs utilize the full range of possibilities for massage (event, maintenance, and rehabilitation). Other programs provide one aspect or another, for example, just recovery after practices, regular maintenance, or only event massage.

Massage in Physical Education and Athletics

By the beginning of the 20th century, massage and exercise were well known in the United States as therapeutic agents. Americans who had studied at the Central Institute in Stockholm and Swedish immigrants first brought Pehr Ling's systems of educational and medical gymnastics to the United States in the 1850s. Ling's medical gymnastics were popularly known in the United States as the Swedish movement cure, a system of restoring health through active and passive movements. Passive movements included various forms of soft tissue manipulation and passive joint movements. Ling's system found its way into both physical medicine and physical education.

Dio Lewis's Normal Institute of Physical Culture offered instruction in the Swedish movement cure as early as 1862. Hartvig Nissen and Baron Nils Posse, both prominent in the history of physical education, were also practitioners of the Swedish movement cure. Nissen, who arrived in Washington, DC, in 1893 to serve as Vice-Consul from Sweden, opened the Swedish Health Institute for the Treatment of Chronic Diseases by Swedish Movements and Massage (Nissen, 1889).

Classic Western massage, as developed by Johann Metzger (1839–1909) of Amsterdam, was synthesized with the Swedish movements late in the 19th century to create an eclectic system. That system, combined with hydrotherapy, became popularly known as Swedish massage.

Baron Nils Posse also opened a school, the Posse Normal School of Physical Education in Boston, that maintained clinics in several large Boston hospitals and where in the 1890s medical gymnastics and massage were taught. Graduates of the Posse program were trained in both educational and medical gymnastics, modeling Ling's Royal Institute of Gymnastics in Stockholm.

In 1915 R. Tait McKenzie, an MD and a professor of physical education, published the second edition of *Exercise in Education and Medicine*, which examined the role of exercise in physical education, recreation, athletics, and rehabilitation. These fields were not clearly distinguished then, and practitioners trained in one area often worked in a related field.

Many reconstruction aides who used massage, Swedish movements, and hydrotherapy to rehabilitate soldiers wounded in World War I were trained in schools of physical education. In 1928 Stafford wrote, "The branches of physiotherapy which have been and will continue to be handled by physical educators are those of massage and therapeutic exercise and certain phases of heat and water treatments" (p. xiii).

This tradition continued to the 1950s, physical education programs serving as the training grounds for physical therapists. Athletic training still has vestiges of this connection to physiotherapy, as do a small number of kinesiotherapy programs within U.S. physical education departments. It is not surprising that massage would be part of training athletes in schools and universities. Most likely an ancient tradition of massage for athletes, passed down informally through trainers, was enriched by new developments in therapeutic massage and merged into physical education (as the specialty of athletic massage) in the early 20th century.

McKenzie (1915) speaks of trainers commonly knowing the benefits of athletic massage:

> Its action in improving muscle tone, in postponing the onset of fatigue and hastening recovery from it, has long been recognized by athletic trainers. In preparing athletes for a contest, general massage is always given by friction, kneading, pinching, and stroking, lubricating the surface with some oily liniment. After a hard race or other contest it is a matter of common knowledge among trainers that a five-minute treatment will enable an athlete to repeat or continue a performance otherwise impossible. (p. 340)

Given this heritage, it seems natural that sports massage is again finding a welcome place in school athletic departments across the United States.

A Master Schedule

Ideally, the full team of sports professionals (e.g., coach, athletic trainer, athletic department, and the sports massage specialist) develops a master schedule for sports massage. The master schedule will be altered as the season progresses and schedules shift, athletes develop certain needs, and other factors change.

Developing a master schedule of sports massage sessions takes into consideration practice and nonpractice days, time available before and after practices, and time around competitions. Other factors to consider include duration and frequency of the sessions and space available.

A session's duration depends on its proximity to competition, time available, and objectives to be accomplished and will vary with each situation. Blocks of time can be set aside for sports massage, and the sessions within that block can be planned on the actual day of the sessions.

Scheduling massage for team sports presents more of a challenge than for individual sports. For example, basketball, football, field hockey, and soccer teams tend to warm up as a team whereas the pre-event preparation for individual sports tends to be more solitary. Pre-event massage for the whole team may not make much sense; however, individuals on a team may benefit from pregame massage. Recovery and maintenance massage can be scheduled over a longer period of time and can be given regularly after and between games.

Instructing athletes in self-massage and partner massage might also be part of the master plan. Coaches might want their own workshop on using massage with their athletes. Figure 7.1 shows a sample master schedule for a track team.

	Sunday	Monday	Tuesday	Wednesday	Thursday	Friday	Saturday
	Rest day	Practice	Practice SMS*—1/2-hour maintenance sessions	Practice Workshop on partner and self-massage	Practice	Travel Short practice SMS—1/2-hour sessions in preparation for meet	All-day meet SMS—pre-, inter, and postevent sessions
	Rest day	Practice	Practice SMS—1/2-hour maintenance sessions	Practice	Local meet SMS—pre-, inter, and postevent sessions	Short practice SMS—1/2-hour recovery sessions	Practice
	Rest day	Practice	Practice SMS—1/2-hour maintenance sessions	Practice	Practice	Travel Short practice SMS—1/2-hour sessions in preparation for meet	Weekend meet SMS—pre-, inter, and postevent sessions
	Weekend meet SMS—pre-, inter, and postevent sessions	Short practice	Practice SMS—1/2-hour maintenance sessions	Practice	Practice	Practice	Local meet SMS—pre-, inter, and postevent sessions

*SMS = Sports massage specialist

Figure 7.1
Sample 4-week master sports massage schedule for a track team.

Space and Equipment

Ideally, a special room for massage is set aside, but the space can be improvised in a training room, locker room, or office.

Massage specialists may travel with the teams to important competitive events. On the road, a hotel room can be set up for massage. Frequently at individual sport competitions, a space is set aside at the event site for massage. You should check with the event planners in advance to see if they have provided suitable space.

Massage specialists often have their own equipment, but you may want to provide a portable massage table or special massage chair for events away from home. A tent or other shelter is often used at outdoor events as a shield from sun and rain as shown in Figure 7.2.

Supplies may be provided by the event coordinator or sponsoring school, or some may be brought by sports massage specialists themselves. These supplies include

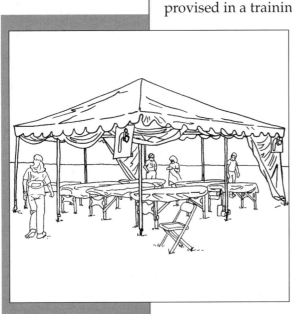

Figure 7.2
Shelter for sports massage at outdoor events.

- a plastic fitted sheet to protect the massage table;

- alcohol solution to wipe the table clean between athletes;

- paper towels to wipe tables and clean hands between sessions;

- a garbage bag for paper towels;

- blankets, space blankets, and head and hand coverings for athletes with hypothermia;

- water for fluid replacement and warm broth in cold weather;

- ice and baggies and ice cups;

- bleach solution (1 part bleach to 10 parts water) or other disinfectant and latex gloves (see Appendix A for situations in which blood is present);

- sunscreen, a hat, bug spray, and snacks (for personal comfort as appropriate in outdoor situations); and

- miscellaneous useful items such as spray bottles, cotton towels, masking tape, and a clipboard and paper for signing in athletes.

Finding the Resources

How do you find a sports massage specialist? Look for graduates of massage training programs that include sports massage as a specialty or locate a massage therapist who has taken continuing education courses in sports massage. Some local professional associations for massage therapists have teams that provide pre-event and postevent massage for amateur competitions; they might also have lists of available specialists. The

National Sports Massage Team of the American Massage Therapy Association can also provide names of persons who have passed a certification examination in sports massage for pre-event and postevent work. (Call or write the National Sports Massage Team at the American Massage Therapy Association, 820 Davis St., Suite 100, Evanston, IL 60201-4444, 708-864-0123 for more information.)

In school and university programs with tight budgets, funding a massage specialist may be a challenge. Funds may come from the regular athletic budget or from outside sources. In some cases, a booster club for a school or specific team provides funds for a sports massage program.

Massage specialists often work on contract and are usually paid by the hour or by the session. They may also be employees of an athletic organization, similar to athletic trainers. Responsible students can be trained as assistant massage specialists, much like student trainers. They might work under the supervision of a sports massage specialist, a coach, or an athletic trainer.

Just as the athletic trainer should be available to all students, in an ideal situation the sports massage program should serve all athletes. To accomplish this, several professional massage specialists can be hired, student assistants trained, self-massage and partner massage can be taught, or some combination of the preceding can be implemented. Student interns from a local massage school are another possible resource. With a firm commitment, good planning, and a little creativity, resources for a sports massage program can be found.

Training Athletes and Coaches to Give Massage

Your state or local government may require a license to practice massage, although some laws exempt those working with athletic teams. Appendix B lists the addresses of state licensing authorities for states that require licensing of massage practitioners.

Athletes can learn to do self-massage and partner massage for a variety of situations including warm-ups, preactivity and postactivity, and general maintenance. An experienced sports massage specialist can teach simple and effective no-oil massage techniques in a workshop. With some follow-up supervision, this should be sufficient to start athletes giving massages to themselves and each other (King, 1993).

In addition, coaches may want their own workshop to learn how they can use massage to enhance their coaching. Because of their special relationship to athletes, coaches might use massage differently, for example, when giving last minute instructions before a performance or for psychological effect.

PROFESSIONAL AND ELITE AMATEUR ATHLETES

Many professional and elite amateur athletes hire their own sports massage specialists. This is especially true in individual sports like tennis, running, boxing, and cycling where the athletes have their own choice of coaches, athletic trainers, personal physicians, and other support staff. Sometimes tournament managers (e.g., on a professional tennis circuit) provide a massage specialist for all players. Or an Olympic team may have its own massage specialist who travels with the team to training camp and to the games.

Some professional sport teams hire a team massage specialist to provide massage to all team members. This assures that players will at least receive regular recovery massage, maintenance massage, or both. The logistics for providing massage in the circumstances mentioned above are similar to schools and universities, that is, scheduling, space, equipment, and travel.

ORGANIZED ATHLETIC EVENTS

One of the most publicly recognized settings for sports massage today is at organized athletic events. Teams of sports massage specialists are visible at such prestigious events as the Olympic Games, Pan-American Games, Goodwill Games, and the Boston Marathon. They are also found at regional and local 10K and fun runs and school track and swim meets.

A sports massage team is typically composed of several massage specialists who provide massage for competitors at the event. Event organizers commonly view sports massage as either a separate service or a part of the medical team. Corporate sponsors may fund sports massage teams.

Sports massage at these events differs from other settings because here a massage specialist is most often working on strangers and for a limited period of time—sometimes as little as 15 minutes each. Postevent massage might also involve first aid and recognizing signs of more serious problems that need to be referred to the medical team. Postevent massage needs to be well coordinated.

General Guidelines for Sports Massage Teams

There are some general guidelines for organizing a sports massage team for an event.

- Establish criteria for sports massage team members (e.g., training and experience).

- Plan and implement recruitment of massage practitioners who meet criteria well in advance of the event.

- Arrange for funding via the general event budget or corporate sponsor. Get agreements in writing.

- Clearly define the scope of responsibility for the sports massage team and its relationship to other staff members, especially the medical team.

- Arrange for orientation of massage practitioners close to the event time to go over logistics.

- Meet with event organizers to review the logistics of providing sports massage (e.g., how many athletes are expected, how many massage sessions will be given, will a shelter be provided, who provides supplies, what are the hours, arrangement of tables).

- Organize the massage operation (e.g., traffic flow in massage area, processing athletes [intake forms], assignment of athletes to specialists, assistants).
- Address other concerns (e.g., parking, breaks, timing sessions).

Coordinate With the Medical Team

Ideally, the sports massage team at an organized athletic event coordinates its work with the event's medical team. Some suggestions for event organizers follow:

- Develop a protocol for referral of injured athletes from the massage area to the medical area.
- Establish a clear path for movement between the two areas.
- Station someone from the medical team in the sports massage area to handle emergencies.
- Station some experienced massage specialists in the medical area to help with situations in which massage is most beneficial.

THE ATHLETE'S SUPPORT TEAM

What is the place of the sports massage specialist in relation to other members of the athlete's support team? Traditionally, massage specialists have a broad range of functions from health maintenance to preparation for events and recovery afterward to remedial and rehabilitation work. Ideally sports massage specialists should be part of the athlete's total support network in which there is a system of interaction and communication among the professionals who care for the same athletes.

In one model of interaction and communication among sport professionals, the "comprehensive" model, the athlete's support team interacts within two concentric circles.

The inner circle represents professionals who focus on enhancing performance, and the outer circle represents team members who treat injuries. A dynamic relationship among the components of the system and frequent coordinated communication and interaction are essential for the model to work most effectively.

Inner Circle

The innermost circle of interaction consists of those concerned specifically with performance enhancement, injury prevention, and addressing minor injuries and complaints: the coach, the athletic trainer, and the massage specialist.

In the early 20th century, a single person, called the "trainer," performed the functions of three sport professionals. Since the mid-20th century, specialists began to perform different aspects of the trainer's work. We now rely on a team of trainers, each focusing on a particular aspect or method of preparing athletes for sport performance. Given this history, it is not surprising to find an overlap of functions.

Generally speaking, coaches focus on the actual performance of the sport and physical conditioning. Athletic trainers assess, treat, and rehabilitate injuries. Sports massage specialists focus on recovery, preparation for competition, and minor problem conditions. All are concerned with injury prevention.

Massage has traditionally been used to prepare athletes for the physical exertion of training sessions and competition, and especially for recovery afterward. This aspect of sports massage focuses on the healthy athlete and the enhancement of normal physical and mental functioning.

As mentioned previously, the trained massage specialist can often detect abnormalities in tissues, joint movement, and psychological conditions—before they cause deterioration of performance or debilitating pain. The massage specialist can alert the coach and athletic trainer to potential problem conditions so they can modify the athlete's training accordingly. Maintenance massage can address problem areas and restore conditions to a more normal state before they become chronic problems or acute injuries.

Massage specialists may also address minor injuries and complaints, such as tight or sore muscles, and refer athletes with more serious conditions to the athletic trainer.

The athletic trainer typically evaluates complaints, gives first aid, and does preventive taping to minimize the chance of injury or reinjury and for rehabilitation. The trainer may refer some rehabilitation to massage specialists in cases where massage can be most beneficial.

Outer Circle

When an athlete's condition or complaint requires further care or evaluation, interaction and communication move to the outer circle. The intermediary is most often the athletic trainer. Typically, the coach and the massage therapist will refer problem conditions and complaints to the athletic trainer. The athletic trainer, in turn, will refer athletes to the team physician or other appropriate health care providers.

Once the condition is diagnosed and a rehabilitation program is planned, the athlete may receive rehabilitation from a sport physical therapist and often returns to the innermost circle for rehabilitation by the athletic trainer and sometimes by the massage specialist. The athletic trainer is typically the primary coordinator for rehabilitation and is in contact with the team physician.

The involvement of massage specialists in rehabilitation varies with the situation and their training in medical massage. Massage facilitates soft tissue healing and the formation of healthy scar tissue, and massage can help keep the rest of the body healthy while the injured area is healing. Massage may also provide psychological benefits related to feeling cared for.

If the skills of massage specialists are to be fully utilized, the specialists must interact with the coach and athletic trainer on a regular and ongoing basis. In a comprehensive program, athletes would also receive maintenance sports massage regularly, at least weekly, and before and after competitions. The massage specialist would be familiar with the athletes, their sports, and their physical and emotional conditions. They would be able to note changes in the athletes, and tailor their sessions to the athletes' immediate and long-term needs.

THE HEALTH CLUB

Most health clubs offer massage (for a fee) to their members, both fitness buffs and amateur athletes. Scheduling massage is primarily the athlete's personal responsibility. The massage program manager makes sure massage practitioners are available at popular times (e.g., after classes or local competitions).

Well-run health club businesses will make sure the athletes know about the benefits of massage. Marketing massage services might include flyers, bulletin board displays, lectures, and short talks during activity classes. The more knowledgeable about massage other staff persons like personal trainers and teachers are, the more likely they will be to recommend it to their students and clients.

The sports massage specialist may confer with aerobics instructors and personal trainers to better serve mutual clients. A massage specialist may, with further training, double as a personal trainer.

When setting up a massage program at a health club, it is best to plan a massage room or rooms with easy access to the locker rooms. This makes dressing easier and gives better access to showers, steam rooms, sauna, whirlpool, or other typical locker-room amenities. It also helps to find a relatively quiet place—below the aerobics studio or next to the racquetball courts or weight room might be too noisy for a relaxing massage.

If a number of massage specialists are involved, a massage program coordinator or manager can plan schedules, keep records, and take care of other administrative details. Massage specialists usually work on contract, and program managers must be careful to follow IRS guidelines for contract labor.

THE SPORTS MASSAGE CLINIC

Many sports massage specialists maintain private practices in their own offices or clinics. Much like the health club situation, they have to educate potential athlete clients and advertise their services. Working on sports massage teams for organized events or giving talks at local sports clubs are excellent ways to meet potential clients.

In the absence of a ready-made health care system such as in the school team situation, individual sports massage specialists may develop their own system of referrals and communication with coaches, personal trainers, physicians, chiropractors, and other health care professionals who work with athletes.

APPENDIX A

UNIVERSAL PRECAUTIONS FOR SPORTS MASSAGE AT EVENTS

Universal precautions are intended to prevent transmission of serious communicable diseases, such as HIV, hepatitis B, and other blood-borne pathogens. Although sports massage specialists are generally at low risk for contact with blood-borne pathogens, the probability of coming into contact with blood increases while working at sports events. Chafing, blood blisters on the feet, and road rash from falls are all common occurrences at road races, triathlons, and bicycle events.

The following is a summary of universal precautions for sports massage specialists working at sports events:

 1. Use protective barriers, such as latex gloves, to prevent contact with blood, body fluids containing visible blood, or other body fluids to which universal precautions apply.* When removing gloves, take them off inside out; wash hands with bleach solution.

2. If you come into contact with blood or other body fluids that can transmit disease, use these precautions:

   a. Wash hands with a bleach solution of 1 part bleach to 10 parts water.

   b. Immediately and thoroughly wash the table and other surfaces that have had contact with the fluid.

*Universal precautions *do apply* to certain body fluids with which massage specialists are not likely to come in contact (i.e., blood, semen and vaginal/cervical secretions, urine, feces, and vomit). Universal precautions *do not apply* to the following fluids, unless they contain visible blood, because the risk of transmission of disease is extremely low or nonexistent: nasal secretions, saliva, sweat, tears, sputum.

c. Put all waste materials (e.g., paper towels) into a separate plastic bag. This may be considered medical waste, and it should be disposed of properly. Check with medical personnel at the event site for proper protocol.

3. Take care to prevent injuries when using sharp instruments or, more common for sports massage specialists, when in the medical area where sharp instruments (e.g., needles) are being used.

For more information see Porth, Carol M. (1994). *Pathophysiology: Concepts of altered health states* (4th ed., pp. 286-287).

APPENDIX B

STATES THAT REQUIRE LICENSING OF MASSAGE PRACTITIONERS*

State licensing laws for massage practitioners often exempt other health professionals from the licensing requirement, for example, nurses, physical therapists, athletic trainers, and others who work with athletes.

Arkansas
  Arkansas Board of Massage Therapy
  P.O. Box 34163
  Little Rock, AR 72203-4163
  501-682-9170

Connecticut
  Connecticut Massage Therapy Inquiries
  Department of Public Health
  150 Washington St.
  Hartford, CT 06106
  203-566-1284

Delaware
  Delaware Massage or Bodywork Practitioners
  Division of Professional Regulation
  O'Neill Bldg.
  P.O. Box 1401
  Dover, DE 19903
  302-739-4522

*Some municipalities in areas without statewide licensing require local licensing for massage practitioners, and local business and zoning laws may restrict massage businesses.

Florida
  Florida Department of Professional Regulation
  Board of Massage
  1940 N. Monroe St.
  Tallahassee, FL 32399-0774
  904-488-6021

Hawaii
  Department of Commerce and Consumer Affairs
  Professional and Vocational Licensing Division
  P.O. Box 3469
  Honolulu, HI 96801
  808-586-2696

Iowa
  Iowa Massage Therapy Advisory Board
  Bureau of Professional Licensing
  Department of Public Health
  Lucas State Office Bldg., 4th Floor
  321 E. 12th St.
  Des Moines, IA 50319-0075
  515-242-5937

Louisiana
  Louisiana Board of Massage Therapists
  P.O. Box 65324
  Baton Rouge, LA 70896
  504-844-0435

Maine
  Maine Department of Professional and Financial Regulation
  Division of Licensing and Enforcement
  Massage Therapists
  State House Station #35
  Augusta, ME 04333
  207-624-8603

Nebraska
  Nebraska Bureau of Examining Boards
  Department of Health
  P.O Box 95007
  Lincoln, NE 68509-5007
  402-471-2115

New Hampshire
  New Hampshire Department of Public Health
  Bureau of Health Facilities Administration
  6 Hazen Dr.
  Concord, NH 03301
  603-271-4592

New Mexico
  New Mexico Board of Massage Therapy
  P.O. Box 25101
  Santa Fe, NM 87504
  505-827-7013

New York
   New York State Education Department
   Division of Professional Licensing Services
   Massage Unit, Rm. 3000
   Cultural Education Center
   Albany, NY 12230
   518-474-3866
   For handbook 518-474-3817

North Dakota
   North Dakota Massage Board
   22 Fremont Dr.
   Fargo, ND 58103-5057
   701-235-9208 or 701-237-4036

Ohio
   Ohio State Medical Board
   77 South High St., 17th Floor
   Columbus, OH 43266-0315
   614-466-3934

Oregon
   Oregon Board of Massage Technicians
   800 NE Oregon St., Ste. 407
   Portland, OR 97232
   503-731-4064

Rhode Island
   Rhode Island Department of Health
   Division of Professional Licensing
   Room 104
   Three Capitol Hill
   Providence, RI 02908-5097
   401-277-2827

Texas
   Texas Massage Therapy Registration Program
   Texas Department of Health
   1100 W. 49th St.
   Austin, TX 78756-3183
   512-834-6616

Utah
   Utah Department of Commerce
   Division of Occupational and Professional Licensing
   160 E. 300 South, 4th Floor
   P.O. Box 45805
   Salt Lake City, UT 84145-0805
   801-530-6628

Washington
   Washington Department of Health
   Health Professions Quality Assurance Division
   P.O. Box 47868
   Olympia, WA 98504-7868
   206-586-6351

GLOSSARY

adhesion—A binding together of two anatomical surfaces that are normally separate. Occurs frequently in muscle and connective tissue after trauma or with chronic tension. Deep-transverse friction is used to break up adhesions.

beating—A percussion massage technique applied with a lightly closed fist using the hypothenar eminence and small finger as the striking surface; used for stimulation.

broadening—A massage technique in which muscle and fascial tissue are compressed and broadened with a deep, slow, sliding motion; used to break adhesions and increase circulation.

circular friction—A friction massage technique applied in a circular motion covering no more than 1 square inch at a time; used to break adhesions and for specific warming.

compression—A massage technique that employs a gradual compressing of tissue followed by a gradual reduction of pressure; used to increase circulation. See *palmar compression* and *digital compression*.

contract/relax—An active movement used to promote muscular relaxation through consciously tensing and then relaxing a specific muscle or muscle group.

contract/relax/stretch—A technique used to enhance stretching by preceding the stretch with contract/relax of the muscle to be lengthened.

cupping—A percussion massage technique applied with "cupped" hands (i.e., fingers pressed together with no palm contact); used for stimulation.

debility—A condition that reduces or hinders the athlete's ability to perform his or her sport, but is not totally disabling. See *remedial*.

deep friction—Massage techniques that utilize short, circular, or back-and-forth motions applied with the fingertip or thumb and using sufficient pressure to produce motion on the tissues beneath the skin; used to treat a specific small area and prevent adhesions.

deep-transverse friction—A friction massage technique applied in a direction across the length of the muscle fibers using heavy pressure; used to break adhesions.

digital compression—A compression massage technique applied with the thumb or fingertips; used in various kinds of point work (e.g., trigger point, acupressure point, stress point).

disability—A condition that does not allow athletes to perform their sport at all. See *rehabilitation*.

durable hyperemia—Hyperemia that lasts for a long period of time; one of the goals in pre-event massage. Compression and broadening techniques are often used to induce durable hyperemia. See *hyperemia*.

effleurage—A classic Western massage term for *sliding movements*; found in Swedish and Russian massage.

event massage—An application of sports massage in the time period surrounding a competitive event that aims at immediate performance enhancement, recovery, or both. Includes pre-event, interevent, and postevent massage.

general relaxation—Physiological state characterized by decreases in heart rate, oxygen consumption, respiration, and skeletal muscular activity and by increases in skin resistance and alpha brain waves; sometimes called the relaxation response.

hacking—A percussion massage technique applied with the little, third, and fourth fingers with the palms facing each other; used for stimulation.

hyperemia—Increased blood flow to part of the body. Massage techniques used to induce hyperemia include deep sliding strokes, kneading, and compression.

hypertonicity—Increase in muscle tone resulting in muscle tension.

hypoxia—Insufficient amount of oxygen.

interevent—A type of event massage given in the short periods between events in an extended competition that aims at recovery from one performance and preparation for optimal performance in the next event.

ischemia—Insufficient blood flow to tissue that results in a decreased oxygen supply (hypoxia), increased carbon dioxide, and an insufficient supply of nutrients. Can cause pain, stiffness, and soreness in the affected area.

jostling—A massage technique in which the soft tissues are shaken back and forth with short, quick, loose movements; may be accompanied by mobilization of surrounding joints; used to loosen up an area.

kneading—A massage movement in which the hands alternately and rhythmically lift, squeeze, and release the soft tissues; used for muscular relaxation and increasing circulation in the tissues.

maintenance—An all-purpose application of sports massage that is scheduled between competitions. It aims at recovery, normalizing stressed tissues, and treating minor injuries and complaints.

massage—The manipulation of the soft tissues of the body.

massage specialist—A person with special skills in massage and related techniques, gained through education and experience.

massage therapist—A specialist in massage therapy who has graduated from an approved or accredited training program and who, in some states, holds an occupational license as a massage therapist.

muscular relaxation—Opposite of a state of contraction in skeletal muscles. A reduction in muscle hypertonicity, induced by massage techniques including sliding strokes, kneading, vibration, and jostling.

muscle tension—State of hypertonicity in skeletal muscle usually caused by stress, trauma, or overuse.

palmar compression—A compression massage technique applied with the palm of one hand while hands are in the palmar-overlay position; used to increase circulation to a broad area.

percussion—Massage techniques that employ a rapid, rhythmic hitting movement applied with the hands or fingertips. See *beating, cupping, hacking, pincement, slapping, tapping*. Same as *tapotement*.

petrissage—A classic Western massage term for *kneading*; found in Swedish and Russian massage.

pincement—A percussion massage technique applied with the thumb and fingers in rapid, light, lifting movements on the skin; used for stimulation.

postevent—A type of event massage given after a competition. It aims at recovery, treatment of minor injuries and complaints, and responding to health emergencies.

pre-event—A type of event massage given from 4 hours to up to 1/2 hour before competition. It aims at preparing the athlete in mind and body for optimal performance.

proprioceptive neuromuscular facilitation (PNF)—A method of promoting or hastening the response of the neuromuscular mechanism to relax or lengthen a muscle through stimulation of the proprioceptors. See *contract–relax, contract–relax–stretch, reciprocal inhibition*.

range of motion (ROM)—The degree of movement of a joint before the movement is impinged upon by surrounding tissues; active or passive movement of a joint through its range of motion for evaluative or therapeutic purposes.

reciprocal inhibition—A physiological phenomenon in which an opposing muscle group (antagonist) relaxes when the agonist group contracts; sometimes used with a stretch of antagonist muscles.

recovery—Application of sports massage after strenuous workouts and competitions to assist the athlete in regaining optimal physical and mental condition and reducing the harmful effects of stress.

rehabilitation—Application of sports massage aimed at restoring an athlete to normal or near-normal function after a disabling injury.

remedial—Application of sports massage to treat conditions that reduce or hinder the athlete's ability to perform his or her sport, but that are not disabling. See *debility*.

restoration—Restoring an athlete to optimal condition from a state of stress, debility, or disability; includes recovery, remedial, and rehabilitation applications of massage; in Russian literature often means recovery only.

rocking—A joint mobilization technique in which a body part is moved rhythmically from side to side or back and forth; may accompany jostling or compression.

session—Application of massage within a specific time period, having a beginning, middle, and end and specific goals. Examples from sports massage include a maintenance session and a postevent session.

slapping—A percussion massage technique applied with the entire palmar surface of the hands or pads of fingers with light slapping movements; often used for stimulation.

sliding movements—Massage techniques that use a sliding motion (i.e., hands move across the skin with even pressure and a broad contact surface); used to apply lubricants, for warming and preparing an area for deeper massage, for general relaxation, and as a connecting or concluding technique.

sports massage—The application of massage therapy to athletes and others engaged in intense physical activity for performance enhancement and health maintenance. Sports massage is commonly used for conditioning, recovery, remediation of problem conditions, and rehabilitation; may be scheduled pre-event, interevent, or postevent or between competitions and tournaments.

tapotement—A classic Western massage term for *percussion* techniques; found in Swedish and Russian massage.

tapping—A percussion massage technique applied with the fingertips or finger pads and typically used in delicate areas such as the face and head; used for stimulation.

thixotrophy—A property of soft tissues by which they become more fluid after movement or when stirred up and more rigid when immobile.

thumb slide—A massage technique applied with the outer side of the thumb using a sliding motion to compress muscle and fascial tissue.

treatment—Application of massage for a specific purpose that may include wellness, remediation, or rehabilitation.

vibration—A massage technique in which the hand or fingertips create a trembling motion.

wellness—A dynamic state of health in which a person strives for optimal body–mind functioning.

REFERENCES

Alter, M.J. (1990). *Sport stretch*. Champaign, IL: Leisure Press.

Anderson, B. (1980). *Stretching*. Bolinas, CA: Shelter.

Anderson, K.N., & Anderson, L.E. (1990). *Mosby's pocket dictionary of medicine, nursing, & allied health*. St. Louis: Mosby.

Anshel, M.H. (1991). *Dictionary of the sport and exercise sciences*. Champaign, IL: Human Kinetics.

Arnheim, D.D., & Prentice, W.E. (1993). *Principles of athletic training* (8th ed.). St. Louis: Mosby Yearbook.

Baumgartner, A.J. (1947). *Massage in athletics*. Minneapolis: Burgess.

Bell, A.J. (1964). Massage and the physiotherapist. *Physiotherapy*, **50**, 406-408.

Benjamin, P.J. (1993). Unpublished interview with Jill Bielawski, massage therapist for the University of Arizona swim team, September 2, 1993.

Birukov, A.A., & Peisahov, N.M. (1979). Changes in the psychophysiological indices using different techniques of sports massage. *Teoriya i Praktika Fizicheskoi Kultury*, **8**, 21-24. Translated in M. Yessis (Ed.) (1986) *Soviet Sports Review*, **21**, 1, 29.

Birukov, A.A., & Pogosyan, M.M. (1983). Special means of restoration of work capacity of wrestlers in the periods between bouts. *Teoriya i Praktika Fizicheskoi Kultury*, **3**, 49-50. Translated in M. Yessis (Ed.) (1983) *Soviet Sports Review*, **19**, 4, 191-192.

Boone, T., Cooper, R., & Thompson, W.R. (1991). A physiologic evaluation of the sports massage. *Athletic Training*, **26**, 51-54.

Bullock, D.M. (1925). *Athletic training methods*. N.p.

Chaitow, L. (1988). *Soft-tissue manipulation*. Rochester, VT: Healing Arts Press.

Crosman, L.J., Chateauvert, S.R., & Weisburg, J. (1985). The effects of massage to the hamstring muscle group on range of motion. *Massage Journal*, 59-62.

Curtis, J.D., Detert, R.A., Schindler, J., & Zirkel, K. (1985). *Teaching stress management and relaxation skills: An instructor's guide*. La Crosse, WI: Coulee Press.

Cyriax, J.H., & Cyriax, P.J. (1993). *Illustrated manual of orthopedic medicine* (2nd ed.). Boston: Butterworth & Heinemann.

Dubrovsky, V.I. (1982). Changes in muscle and venous flow after massage. *Teoriya i Praktika Fizicheskoi Kultury*, **4**, 56-57. Translated in M. Yessis (Ed.) (1980) *Soviet Sports Review*, **18**, 3, 134-135.

Fay, H.J. (1916). *Scientific massage for athletes*. London: Ewart, Seymour.

Field, T., Fox, N., Pickens, J., Ironsong, G., & Scafidi, F. (1993). *Job stress survey*. Unpublished manuscript, Touch Research Institute, University of Miami School of Medicine. (Reported in *Touchpoints: Touch Research Abstracts*, **1**[1], 1993.)

Field, T., Morrow, C., Valdeon, C., Larson, S., Kuhn, C., & Schanberg, S. (1992). Massage reduces anxiety in child and adolescent psychiatric patients. *Journal of the American Academy of Child and Adolescent Psychiatry*, **31**, 1, 125-131.

Frierwood, H.T. (1953, September-October). The place of health service in the total YMCA program. *Journal of Physical Education*, p. 21.

Harmer, P.A. (1991). The effect of pre-performance massage on stride frequency in sprinters. *Athletic Training*, **26**, 55-59.

Johnson, E.L. (n.d.). *The history of YMCA physical education*. Chicago: Association Press.

Johnson, W. (1866). *The anatriptic art*.

Jordan, K.D., & Jessup, D. (1990, Winter). The recuperative effects of sports massage as compared to rest. *Massage Therapy Journal*, pp. 57-67.

Juhan, D. (1987). *Job's body: A handbook for bodywork*. Barrytown, NY: Station Hill Press.

King, R.K. (1993). *Performance massage*. Champaign, IL: Human Kinetics.

Kresge, C.A. (1983). Massage and sports. In O. Appenzeller & R. Atkinson (Eds.), *Sports medicine: Fitness, training, injuries* (pp. 367-380). Baltimore: Urban & Schwarzenberg.

Lamp, S.P. (1989, Spring). Working in the optimal therapy zone. *Massage Therapy Journal*, pp. 24-25.

Matveeva, E.A., & Tsirgiladze, I.V. (1985). Use of underwater steam massage and hydroelectric baths in restoration of boxers (condensed). *Boks*, **1**, 28-29.

McKenzie, R.T. (1915). *Exercise in education and medicine* (2nd ed.). Philadelphia: Saunders.

McSwain, G. (1990). *The effect of massage, exercise, and rest on the clearance rate of blood lactate after strenuous exercise*. Unpublished master's thesis, California State University at Fullerton.

Meagher, J. (1990). *Sportsmassage*. Barrytown, NY: Station Hill Press.

Murphy, M.C. (1914). *Athletic training*. New York: Scribner's.

Namikoshi, T. (1985). *Shiatsu and stretching*. Tokyo: Japan Publications.

Nickel, D.J. (1984). *Acupressure for athletes*. Santa Monica, CA: Health Acu Press.

Nissen, H. (1889). *A manual of instruction for giving Swedish movement and massage treatment*. Philadelphia: Davis.

Pollard, D.W. (1902). *Massage in training*. Unpublished thesis, International Young Men's Christian Association Training School, Springfield, MA.

Sinyakov, A.F., & Belov, E.S. (1982). Restoration of work capacity of gymnasts. *Gymnastika*, **1**, 48-51.

Stafford, G.T. (1928). *Preventive and corrective physical education*. New York: Barnes.

Tappan, F.M. (1988). *Healing massage techniques: Holistic, classic, and emerging methods*. Norwalk, CT: Appleton & Lange.

Tisserand, R.B. (1977). *The art of aromatherapy*. Rochester, VT: Destiny Books.

Travell, J.G., & Simons, D.G. (1983). *Myofascial pain and dysfunction: The trigger point manual*. Baltimore: Williams & Wilkins.

Travell, J.G., & Simons, D.G. (1992). *Myofascial pain and dysfunction: The trigger point manual: The lower extremeties. Vol. 2*. Baltimore: Williams & Wilkins.

Williams, R.J. (1943). Second annual national YMCA health service clinic. *Journal of Physical Education*, **41**, 30.

Workshop on Alternative Medicine. (1994). *Alternative medicine: Expanding medical horizons* (NIH Publication No. 94-066). Washington, DC: U.S. Government Printing Office.

Yackzan, L., Adams, C., & Francis, K.T. (1984). The effect of ice massage on delayed muscle soreness. *American Journal of Sports Medicine*, **12**, 159.

Yates, J. (1990). *A physician's guide to therapeutic massage: Its physiological effects and their application to treatment*. Vancouver, BC: Massage Therapists Association of British Columbia.

Zalessky, M. (1979). Coaching, medico-biological and psychological means of restoration. *Legkaya Atletika*, **7**, 20-22.

Zalessky, M. (1980). Restoration for middle, long-distance, steeplechase and marathon runners and speed walkers. *Legkaya Atletika*, **3**, 10-13.

INDEX

ABOUT THE AUTHORS

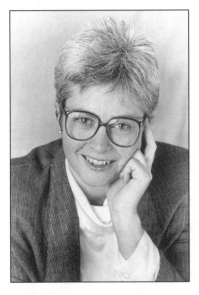

With more than 30 years in health, fitness, physical education, coaching, and massage therapy, **Patricia Benjamin's** varied background offers her special insight into the benefits of massage for athletes.

Benjamin graduated from the Chicago School of Massage Therapy in 1984. She is a licensed massage therapist in Connecticut and nationally certified in therapeutic massage and bodywork. In 1981 she earned her PhD in recreation and leisure studies from Purdue University.

Benjamin serves as the dean and the director of education at the Chicago School of Massage Therapy. She was the national director of education for the American Massage Therapy Association (AMTA) from 1989 to 1993 and owned her own massage business from 1986 until 1990. Benjamin was an assistant professor at the University of Illinois at Chicago in the College of Health, Physical Education, and Recreation for seven years. She also taught physical education and coached at the high school level for seven years.

Benjamin is an active member in the AMTA. She lives in Chicago, Illinois, where she enjoys traveling, antiquing, hiking, martial arts, and researching the history of massage.

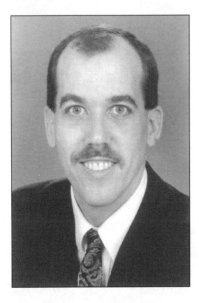

Scott Lamp has been a massage therapist since 1982 and has worked with athletes at all levels. He was the first massage therapist in the United States to be hired by a Division I college athletic association (University of Florida) to provide an ongoing massage therapy program, and he worked there for eight years.

Lamp is now the owner/director of Southeastern Sports Massage, a sports massage clinic that develops and implements a variety of projects and programs. He also has his own private practice that serves more than 30 clients per week ranging from professional athletes and Olympic gold medalists to weekend warriors and gardeners. In addition, he develops and teaches certification courses for sports massage therapy.

Lamp graduated from the Soma School of Massage in Gainesville, Florida, in 1982 and was licensed by the state of Florida the same year. In 1992 he was nationally certified in therapeutic massage and bodywork. He earned his BS in botany from the University of Florida in 1980.

Lamp is past president of the AMTA. In 1991 he was awarded the National Meritorious Award and the Florida Chapter Meritorious Award from the AMTA.

Lamp lives in Gainesville, Florida, and enjoys tennis, travel, and spiritual study.